Marking Off Breast Cancer: Navigating The Journey With Strength, Hope And Awareness

SARA DAVIS

Published by SARA DAVIS, 2024.

While every precaution has been taken in the preparation of this book, the publisher assumes no responsibility for errors or omissions, or for damages resulting from the use of the information contained herein.

MARKING OFF BREAST CANCER: NAVIGATING THE JOURNEY WITH STRENGTH, HOPE AND AWARENESS

First edition. October 21, 2024.

Copyright © 2024 SARA DAVIS.

ISBN: 979-8227359636

Written by SARA DAVIS.

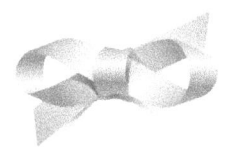

Introduction

The road of breast cancer is one that anyone ever anticipates taking. It brings with it a flurry of feelings, anxieties, and inquiries; it doesn't send out invitations or request permission. It can seem as though the world has abruptly vanished, leaving only uncertainty for anyone receiving a breast cancer diagnosis. How do you start to come to terms with this new reality? Where do you go when you need direction, answers, or hope? When the road ahead becomes overwhelming and you need a guide and a friend, Marking Off Breast Cancer: Navigating the Journey with Strength, Hope, and Awareness is the book for you.

This is an invitation to navigate breast cancer with a combination of information, empathy, and empowerment—it is not just another medical manual or textbook. Breast cancer has an impact on a person's identity, emotions, relationships, and future in addition to their physical health. It necessitates consideration of the mental and physical environments. Although medical care is essential to this process, the trip also requires something more profound—strength in the face of hardship, hope when the future is uncertain, and an understanding that this fight is not waged alone but rather with innumerable others who have traveled a similar path.

This book's title, "Marking Off Breast Cancer," was chosen with purpose. There are milestones at every stage of the journey—diagnosis, treatment, recovery, and survivorship—some of which you expect and some of which come as a surprise. This road is not endless, and these milestones remind us of that. A beginning, middle, and end are all present. Furthermore, although breast cancer may leave its mark, the whole experience need not be defined by it. Every action presents a chance to take back your story, face obstacles head-on, and make decisions with clarity and purpose. As you cross these phases off, you'll discover that, despite its challenges, the road ahead is manageable. A Call to Proceed with Fortitude, Hope, and Consciousness

In the end, empowerment is the main theme of Marking Off Breast Cancer: Navigating the Journey with Strength, Hope, and Awareness. It's about realizing that you have choices about how you choose to take this route, even though you may not have chosen it. This book provides direction, empathy, and useful tools to help you go with confidence, regardless of whether you're just starting the trip, helping a loved one through it, or thinking back on your own experience as a survivor.

Breast cancer is a life experience as much as a medical illness. It alters your perspective on the future, your relationships, and yourself. However, there is space for development, recovery, and a fresh sense of purpose inside that shift. Together, we'll cross off the stages, acknowledge the successes, and confront the obstacles with the knowledge that, despite its effects, breast cancer does not define a person.

Chapter 1

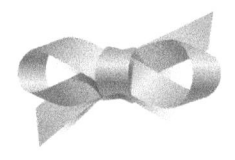

Understanding the Diagnosis

"YOU HAVE BREAST CANCER" can cause a sudden change in reality. The intricacies of those words are frequently not entirely understood at the time. The diagnosis itself is more than simply a name; it's a complex web of medical terminology, feelings, and inquiries that flow through a person's head. It's not only about the illness; it's also about knowing what each stage signifies for your attitude, alternatives, and personal narrative.

There are various types of breast cancer. There isn't a diagnosis that works for everyone. Words like triple-negative breast cancer, invasive ductal carcinoma, ductal carcinoma in situ (DCIS), HER2-positive, and hormone receptor-positive may be strange to you, but they all have meaning. What type is this breast cancer? How combative? Although the intricacy of these classifications may seem intimidating, the confusion begins to clear with time and direction. As you gain more knowledge, these medical phrases become less foreign and start to serve as a guide for making decisions.

In order to educate and enlighten you before treatment decisions are made, doctors and medical personnel frequently work rapidly to explain the biology underlying your diagnosis. Mammograms, biopsies, ultrasounds, and MRI scans are among the diagnostic tools that become a part of your life. Each of these aims to provide a more comprehensive image of your inside surroundings as well as the lump or anomaly. Cancer does not occur in a vacuum. It has an effect on your immune system, hormones, cells, and even your mood. The goal of the diagnostic phase is to determine the extent of the cancer's spread, whether it is contained, and what the future prospects are.

Discussions regarding stages are also prompted by the first diagnosis. While Stage I may seem comforting, Stage IV is much less so. However, these figures don't fully reflect the path ahead. Yes, they are markers, but they don't tell you what to expect from treatment or how your body will react. While some individuals with Stage IV diagnoses live for years, others with early diagnoses may experience an unforeseen amount of upheaval. Stages are markers that aid in framing the course of treatment; they are not guarantees.

There's the emotional aspect to take into account as you begin to grasp the medical jargon. The diagnosis is a trigger for a wide range of emotions rather than only a clinical designation. There can first be a generalized numbness. Shock is a normal reaction. Sometimes the gravity of the problem is too much for the intellect to handle at once. Denial can sometimes creep in as a coping strategy to keep you afloat when reality becomes too much to handle. However, as time passes, this mental haze frequently dissipates and is replaced with feelings of dread, rage, grief, or even resolve. Although each person's reaction is unique, no reaction is incorrect. It's a very intimate experience.

Some people struggle to comprehend the diagnosis, wondering how their body came to be in this state, whether something might have been done sooner, or whether this is an internal betrayal. It is possible to place blame on oneself for failing to recognize the warning signs sooner or on outside variables such as family history, lifestyle decisions, and environmental hazards. It's simple to become caught up in a never-ending cycle of "what ifs," but assigning blame doesn't alter the present; what counts right now is how to go.

During this time, the dynamic of the connection with healthcare experts changes. It can feel alienating to suddenly be treated like a patient with a serious illness rather than just someone going to the doctor for a checkup. Although oncologists, doctors, and nurses all use technical jargon, there are people navigating this maze behind their white coats and data-driven discussions. Gaining their trust becomes crucial. Sometimes you'll need to speak up for yourself, which could include asking additional questions, getting second perspectives, or just slowing down the conversation to properly understand what is being said.

The question of who to notify and how to tell them also comes up. It can be as hard to break the news to loved ones as it is to receive the diagnosis. Seeing their reactions is more important than simply saying, "I have cancer." Everybody has a distinct way of processing stuff. While some could withdraw because they are unable to comprehend the seriousness of the issue, others might provide support right away. These discussions can differ according on the person you are speaking to, and there is no set way to conduct them. While some individuals will only be interested in your mental health, others might require the clinical specifics. You may discover that the folks you feel most comfortable discussing your event with aren't necessarily the ones closest to you.

However, receiving a breast cancer diagnosis carries additional cultural significance. Public perceptions of the illness are shaped by media representations, awareness campaigns, and pink ribbons, but real-life experiences frequently diverge from those representations. Although breast cancer is frequently accompanied by signals of optimism and survival, receiving a diagnosis can feel more uncertain. The gray areas—doubts regarding the efficacy of therapy, recurrence anxieties, and the long-term effects on one's sense of self—are not usually taken into consideration by the public narrative. Even though awareness efforts are beneficial, there is frequently a gap between the glamorous pictures and the personal hardships that people with diagnoses endure.

In a manner that few other experiences can, the diagnosis drives many people to face their mortality. All of a sudden, the future seems precarious. Even with a favorable prognosis, concerns regarding longevity surface. After this, what does life look like? Will it ever feel like normal? There are no simple answers to these existential problems, and they could persist even after treatment and recovery. You cannot go back to who you were before learning of the diagnosis. Not only does your physical appearance and health change, but so do your perceptions of time, relationships, and even your own identity.

Lastly, the diagnosis is a practical and emotional summons to action. Decisions must be made right away: Which course of treatment to take? How can you change your routine to make time for treatments, surgeries, or hospital stays? Then there are the more profound queries, like how to find strength on this path. In this situation, what does hope look like? How can one maintain awareness of the difficulties and minor triumphs encountered during the journey?

It takes time to comprehend the diagnosis. There will be periods of clarity and periods of bewilderment as the process develops over time.

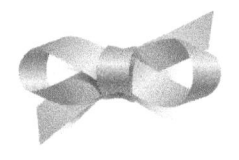

THE DETECTION MOMENT

Everything might change at the moment of discovery, that first moment when something doesn't feel right. Perhaps you start with a self-examination after a standard checkup, a brief sensation, or a mildly bothersome notion. Or maybe it's only an anomaly discovered during a mammogram, a picture that shows something just noticeable but enough to raise an eyebrow. In a series of events, that moment becomes a still frame—powerful but silent, bearing the weight of what lies ahead.

Every woman experiences this moment differently. Some experience numbing denial, while others experience a rush of terror. Confusion frequently arises in the midst of emotional turmoil as people attempt to make sense of how a barely perceptible bump or a shadow on a screen could portend something bigger and more sinister. Time seems to split in this moment, leaving a before and after that characterizes all that happens after. Once it comes to the surface, it cannot be ignored or pushed to the side. It abruptly pushes its way into every nook and cranny of the mind, going from possibility to reality.

It can be similar to being at a threshold with no idea of where to go next, confronted with options and paths that must eventually be followed, but not knowing how to take any of them. It is the first of many steps, each laden with weight and uncertainty, rather than a single one. The once-familiar earth below now feels shaky, as if the fundamental essence of the person is changing suddenly and without permission.

This revelation becomes entwined with the idea of identity. As though viewing it from an unnaturally distanced vantage point, there is a distancing from the life that was known. However, that distance only adds another level of intricacy; it has no effect on the impact. All of a sudden, in spaces where the air feels too heavy and motionless, words like "biopsy," "tumor," and "oncologist" are used. Cancer's lexicon infiltrates even the most private thoughts, serving as indicators of a new reality that needs to be comprehended, even if it initially seems impossible.

Many people associate this moment with waiting. Awaiting the call from the doctor. Awaiting the outcome, awaiting confirmation or rejection of the greatest worries. The mind is always planning scenarios and preparing for news that will permanently alter the path of everyday life during those paused moments. This waiting creates a strange suspension, where people anxiously cling to any semblance of normalcy even though their daily activities seem pointless. Everything that is familiar feels alien, tinted with the possibility of what could be.

Despite the lack of official confirmation, the body also responds. Just knowing that something is wrong causes a physical sensation and an awareness of previously unnoticed places. The skin, the chest, and even the underarms become extremely sensitive, as if the body is aware of it before the mind is really aware of it. In an attempt to maintain a sense of control while embracing vulnerability, this hyperawareness and the unknown combine to produce a precarious balance between terror and control.

However, strength also emerges in this moment. It manifests as a quiet resilience that has been there the entire time, but possibly undetected, rather than as a sudden change or a bold announcement. Making the appointment, asking the proper questions, and demanding to be heard—even when one's mind is racing with doubt—are all tiny acts that build strength. Even when neither wants to, the mind and body adjust. It's a strength that comes from necessity rather than choice, and it's just as strong for it.

Additionally, hope starts to emerge, even though it could seem brittle at first. In other respects, hope walks side by side with fear instead of taking its place. This hope does not entail avoiding the potential consequences or denying what is occurring. It's a silent, unyielding denial that fear alone should rule the environment. Even in the most dire circumstances, hope endures in the little things: the comforting words of a nurse, the confidence of a friend, or the way light streams into a room and provides warmth.

During this period, awareness becomes more acute. The body's understanding, the systems that support it, and the medical advancements that provide options all become more concentrated and clear. This awareness is not passive; it necessitates active participation, understanding how to negotiate the complexities of treatments, viewpoints, and results, as well as knowing what questions to ask and what options are accessible. It's an awareness that necessitates paying close attention to the details, examining, weighing, and taking into account each one.

The connections that surround this event have also changed. Friends, family, and partners all join the story as it develops. While some may fall, unable to handle the demands this trip provides, others may step up in ways that surprise and soothe. Bonds are put to the test, reinforced, and occasionally shattered. As life is seen through a new lens, where time and presence take on new meanings, conversations move from the mundane to the sublime.

By marking out these moments, each with its own significance, the trip shifts from being one discovery to several, each of which reveals something new about the body, the self, relationships, and the surrounding world. Not all of these revelations are disastrous; some reveal hidden depths of connection with others, inner reserves, or unexpected clarity or insight. Each step of this process eliminates control illusions, revealing only what is actual and palpable, and compel self-awareness, which is frequently painful but vitally important.

The outside world could seem far away, as if people traverse it without realizing the profound changes occurring within. Carrying this new reality while the world stays mostly the same can be confusing as you go about your everyday life knowing what's going on behind the surface. However, it also provides a sense of stability—the knowledge that, despite the internal changes, life goes on, providing its own cadence and patterns to observe.

Even if the moment of discovery is crucial, it's just the beginning of a lengthy and frequently convoluted journey. Along the road, one may discover fresh strength, hope, and awareness, but it also carries the weight of the unknown. Although the body and mind may never be the same again, something else may appear as a result of this reshaping—something that wasn't there before but is now unquestionably a part of the trip.

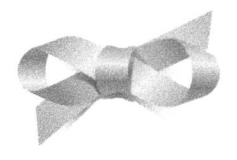

Understanding Medical Phrases

Comprehending medical jargon is essential to the process of diagnosing breast cancer. The key to understanding the complexities of diagnosis, treatment, and overall care is this language, which is frequently complicated. Navigating breast cancer can be a perplexing and overwhelming process if these concepts are not well understood. However, once one learns the terms, a sense of clarity appears, providing knowledge-based empowerment.

The basic words, prefixes, and suffixes that make up medical phrases can resemble a puzzle with their own unique language. Terms like "mammogram," "biopsy," and "mastectomy," for example, are commonly used in the context of breast cancer care and each have important connotations. For instance, a mammography is more than just an X-ray. This low-dose imaging technique was created especially for the breast and aids in the detection of anomalies that might indicate malignancy. When symptoms like lumps are found, it is utilized for both screening and diagnosis.

Another word that comes up when anomalies are discovered is biopsy. A biopsy is more than simply a test; it's a procedure where a tiny piece of tissue is removed to check for the presence of malignant cells. This can be accomplished in a number of ways, including surgical biopsies, which call for a more invasive technique, and needle biopsies, which involve extracting the sample with a tiny needle. Decisions about the next steps in the trip are based on the results of a biopsy.

Words like "stage" and "grade" become crucial if cancer is confirmed. The size of the tumor and whether it has metastasized—or spread to other parts of the body—are factors that determine the stage of breast cancer. Stages I through IV can be used to classify breast cancer; higher numbers denote more advanced illness. The aggressiveness of the cancer is influenced by the grade, which describes how much the malignant cells resemble healthy cells. High-grade malignancies grow and spread more fast than low-grade tumors, which typically grow more slowly.

Medical terminology is further complicated by treatment alternatives. The words "chemotherapy," "radiation," "immunotherapy," and "hormone therapy" are commonly used and each refer to a distinct method of treating the illness. Chemotherapy employs medications to target and kill cancer cells that divide quickly, but it also affects other cells in the body that grow quickly, which can cause typical side effects including fatigue and hair loss. High-energy rays, frequently X-rays, are used in radiation therapy to kill cancer cells in the breast and other locations where the disease has spread.

A relatively recent advancement is immunotherapy, which uses the body's immune system to combat cancer. This treatment either increases the immune response or marks cancer cells so that immune cells can more readily identify them. Contrarily, hormone therapy targets tumors that are stimulated by hormones such as progesterone and estrogen. These medications reduce the hormone levels in the body or prevent these hormones from attaching to cancer cells, which lowers the chance that the cancer will recur.

The experience involves more than just the physical body. The terminology employed also reflects the psychological and emotional toll that breast cancer takes. Words like "survivorship," "remission," and "relapse" have significant emotional connotations in addition to being medical jargon. The period following treatment when a person focuses on their recovery and quality of life while living past their illness is known as "survivorship." Remission may not indicate that cancer is permanently gone, but it does indicate a period of time when the disease is not visible in the body. For many people on this journey, the worry of relapse—the return of cancer after a time of remission—lingers, which is why ongoing monitoring is crucial.

Even the language used to describe breast reconstruction following surgery is unique. A "lumpectomy" involves the removal of a malignant lump while leaving the majority of the breast tissue intact. Mastectomy, on the other hand, entails the whole removal of the breast and frequently leads to discussions regarding choices for reconstruction. Implants or tissue from other areas of the body may be used in reconstruction, and phrases like "flap reconstruction" and "tissue expanders" become commonplace after surgery. These operations involve a very personal decision-making process that frequently necessitates a profound comprehension of the risks, advantages, and anticipated recovery.

Tests and outcomes are crucial in this medical environment. Tests such as "HER2 status," "progesterone receptor (PR) status," and "estrogen receptor (ER) status" establish how the breast cancer may react to therapy. Breast tumors that grow in reaction to progesterone and estrogen are known as PR-positive and ER-positive, respectively. Understanding this can help with hormone therapy decisions. Treatment is also influenced by HER2 status, which refers to a protein that encourages the proliferation of cancer cells. Drugs like trastuzumab that directly target this protein may be beneficial for HER2-positive tumors.

The treatment of breast cancer now includes genetic testing. When talking about inherited risk, phrases like "BRCA1" and "BRCA2" frequently come up. Some people think about preventive treatments like greater surveillance or even prophylactic mastectomy, which involves removing the breast to minimize risk, because mutations in these genes greatly increase the risk of getting breast cancer.

The variety of imaging methods and diagnostic procedures, each with its own unique terminology, is another element that makes the language more difficult to understand. To visualize the breast and surrounding tissues, ultrasound, magnetic resonance imaging (MRI), and computed tomography (CT) scans are frequently used. CT scans employ X-rays, MRIs use magnetic fields and radio waves, and ultrasounds use sound waves to create images. Each is selected according to certain therapeutic demands and offers special advantages of its own.

Clinical trials and newly developed treatments are the subject of additional layers of language. Terms like "randomized controlled trial" (RCT), in which participants are assigned at random to various therapies in order to compare results, may be familiar to patients. Although these trials are essential for creating novel treatments, they also bring with them a new vocabulary and set of considerations, such as the distinction between "standard of care" and "experimental" procedures.

Public awareness campaigns have their own terminology in the broader context of breast cancer advocacy; concepts like "early detection," "self-examination," and "risk factors" are crucial in prevention initiatives. Treatment success is greatly increased by early detection through routine screenings, including mammography. Self-examinations enable people to learn more about their bodies and may help them identify anomalies sooner.

Breast cancer-specific terms and expressions belong to those who are affected by the disease, not merely medical professionals and researchers. By converting the unknown into the intelligible, familiarity with this vocabulary reduces dread by making a confusing deluge of medical information easier to handle. As a result, people dealing with breast cancer can proceed with more resilience, self-awareness, and clarity.

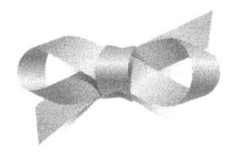

Analyzing the Effect on Emotions

Support becomes crucial as people adjust to this new reality. A vital network of emotional resilience can be established by interacting with loved ones, including family, friends, and even coworkers. Sharing ideas and worries might help people feel less alone and more connected. Support groups or group therapy can provide an environment where people can express themselves without fear of criticism and share stories that have a profound impact on others going through comparable struggles. By reassuring individuals impacted that they are not fighting this battle alone, this shared understanding can foster a feeling of community.

During treatment, the emotional landscape may change significantly. As people gain the ability to speak out for their health and make knowledgeable decisions about their care, a sense of agency frequently develops. Patients can become more empowered by learning more about the illness, turning powerlessness into active participation. A sense of control in the face of uncertainty can be achieved by being knowledgeable about the phases of therapy, possible adverse effects, and the importance of self-care. Every tiny triumph, like finishing a course of chemotherapy or locating a kind medical professional, might be a ray of optimism.

But empowerment also carries the burden of emotional weariness. Physical and emotional exhaustion might result from the demands of treatment plans, doctor's appointments, and the uncertainty of results. As a result of the stress of the diagnosis and treatment, this weariness frequently shows up as worry and despair. It is crucial to acknowledge these emotions, which do not indicate weakness but rather a deep involvement with a transformative event. Many people find comfort in mindfulness exercises that help them develop a sense of presence and serenity, such yoga or meditation.

Coping strategies differ greatly. Some people may find solace in artistic endeavors like writing, painting, or music, which enable them to communicate feelings that are perhaps too nuanced to put into words. Others may turn to nature for comfort, learning that spending time outside may calm the mind and soul. Cooking, gardening, or engaging in hobbies are examples of activities that promote a sense of normalcy and might provide a little reprieve from the demands of therapy.

Opportunities for introspection and reassessing one's priorities in life are also provided by the voyage. Many people say they have a renewed appreciation for the small things in life, including spending time with family, laughing together, and finding some quiet time. This change in viewpoint can give people a fresh sense of purpose by encouraging them to express their values more clearly. Some could decide to take part in advocacy, which involves spreading knowledge about breast cancer and funding support groups or research. By connecting with people who have similar objectives, these acts can turn personal hardships into a source of strength.

The importance of expert assistance in navigating the intricacies of emotions cannot be overstated. Oncology-focused therapists or counselors can provide individualized advice, assisting people in creating unique coping mechanisms for anxiety, bereavement, and the range of emotions that come up during this period. Since physical and mental health are connected in the healing process, addressing emotional health is just as crucial. By promoting resilience and a proactive approach to emotional well-being, incorporating psychological assistance into the care plan can improve the patient's overall quality of life.

As the journey progresses, it becomes clear how important it is to commemorate both tiny and large accomplishments. Every accomplishment is worthy of praise, whether it's finishing treatment, receiving a clean health record, or just feeling better on a particular day. Creating customs around these achievements might help to strengthen resilience and optimism. This could be a private celebration, a get-together with close friends and family, or perhaps just a silent moment of appreciation. These actions not only recognize advancements but also tell a story of resilience and optimism that people can live with.

Navigating uncertainty is a regular struggle in this emotional landscape. Many people remain vigilant due to the uncertainty of health outcomes, which might cause dread of recurrence or new diagnoses. Building a strong toolkit to deal with this unpredictability is essential. Some strategies include letting go of the urge to forecast the future and concentrating on the things that can be managed, like lifestyle decisions, doctor's appointments, and self-advocacy. This accepting process can turn anxiety into a more controllable kind of alertness.

In the end, the human spirit's tenacity is what distinguishes the emotional process of dealing with a breast cancer diagnosis. Every person has a different experience, shaped by their upbringing, networks of support, and coping mechanisms. It takes bravery to embrace vulnerability because it enables people to fully explore their emotions without worrying about being judged. Sharing stories—both happy and sad—creates a tapestry of experiences that speak to people far beyond the individual, increasing awareness and promoting a sense of community.

People frequently discover that hope is a continuous process rather than a single destination when negotiating the emotional toll of this journey. It fluctuates, occasionally coming to the surface suddenly during epiphanies or moments of connection. Despite its difficulties, this path can result in significant personal development and a better comprehension of what it means to live a purposeful life. Every day presents the chance for fresh perspectives and regenerated fortitude, developing a resilience that could alter one's perspective on life and all of its complications.

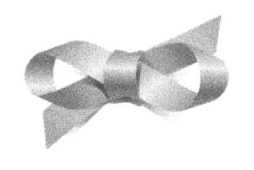

CHAPTER 2:

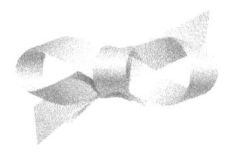

Establishing a Support Network

The voyage rarely occurs alone; rather, it frequently entwines the lives of numerous people. Coping with the physical and mental difficulties that come up can be much improved by knowing how to build this network.

The network of friends and family is the core of any support system. These people are a lifeline because they offer both practical and emotional help. Family members frequently pitch in to help with daily duties like dinner preparation and housework. Their presence can reduce stress, enabling the diagnosed individual to concentrate on their therapy and well-being. During difficult times, friends can act as sounding boards by providing company and a sense of normalcy. Making a connection with them might help them feel included and offer a respite from the frequently stressful medical setting.

Another level of connection is provided via support groups. These organizations provide forums for people to talk about their struggles, anxieties, and victories. They offer a distinct perspective that frequently results from common experiences. Participants can express their emotions in these situations without worrying about being judged. Support groups can help people understand they are not alone in their challenges, whether they are held in person or virtually. This sense of belonging can be a source of resilience and strength, providing helpful guidance and insights into coping mechanisms.

A vital part of the support system is also played by medical experts. Social workers, nurses, and oncologists can offer information about coping strategies, side effects, and available treatments. By responding to inquiries and providing advice that demystifies the course of therapy, they can assist in navigating the healthcare system. Developing a relationship with these experts can result in a more individualized approach to treatment, enabling people to successfully advocate for themselves.

During the trip, emotional well-being is crucial. Processing the wide range of emotions that follow a diagnosis can be greatly aided by mental health specialists. Through therapy, people can express their experiences and explore emotions like fear, rage, and sadness in a safe environment. Additionally, mental health professionals can provide coping mechanisms that are customized for each person. In addition to promoting emotional resilience, this method gives patients the skills they need to cope with stress while undergoing treatment.

Practical resources are crucial for navigating this path in addition to emotional help. Breast cancer-related organizations can offer everything from financial aid to educational materials. Many provide services like insurance claim assistance or transportation to assist people in handling the practical aspects of treatment. By using these resources, people can lessen their load and concentrate on their recovery.

Taking care of oneself during this process might also improve general wellbeing. Even in moderation, promoting physical activity can improve mood and give people a sense of control. In addition to fostering social contacts, practices like yoga or light stretching can help people relax and feel less anxious. Nutrition is also important; eating a balanced diet will help you recuperate and feel more energized. Getting advice from a nutritionist can enable people to make knowledgeable dietary decisions.

Including spiritual activities in the network of support might be even more consoling. Some think that spirituality gives them a sense of purpose and serenity, enabling them to find meaning in the midst of adversity. This could entail practicing awareness, meditation, or prayer. By fostering emotional recovery and mental clarity, these activities can help people center themselves in a way that enhances other types of support.

It is essential to speak up for oneself and other members of the support system. Giving people the ability to express their needs guarantees that they get the assistance and attention they need. Beyond individual experiences, this activism can help raise awareness and educate others about breast cancer. Participating in fundraising activities or community gatherings can foster a feeling of connection and purpose, enabling people to make constructive contributions despite their difficulties.

It can also be transformative to include creativity in the support path. Painting, writing, or music are all forms of artistic expression that can be used as a way to release emotions. These artistic pursuits can assist people in processing their experiences and expressing emotions that might be challenging to communicate verbally. By promoting understanding and connection, sharing these works of art with others helps strengthen the support network.

Throughout the trip, it's critical to keep the lines of communication open with loved ones. Building trust and strengthening relationships can be achieved by promoting open communication about emotions, anxieties, and expectations. Establishing routine check-ins with loved ones can be beneficial as it provides an opportunity to share feelings and experiences. Additionally, by reminding people that help is accessible, these exchanges might lessen feelings of loneliness.

It is impossible to ignore the importance of humor in coping. Laughter may be a very effective way to reduce stress and build relationships. Having fun with loved ones might offer a much-needed break from the seriousness of the circumstance. Whether it's through a favorite program, dinners together, or just lighthearted conversation, finding happiness in the little things may add optimism to the journey.

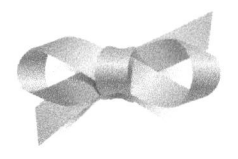

Friends, family, and caregivers

It is common for family members to take up the role of primary caretakers out of obligation and love. They take on the role of advocates, frequently going to appointments with patients and learning complicated medical information with them. By strengthening family ties, this shared pain can turn the experience from an individual hardship into a journey. A close family member's presence can give the patient a sense of security and encourage them to talk more freely about their worries and fears.

Conversely, friends frequently act as a lifeline, bringing happiness and normalcy into the patient's life. Getting together with friends for a laid-back get-together, a movie night, or just a meaningful talk can be a very uplifting experience. The emotional burden associated with receiving a cancer diagnosis is lessened by these encounters, which act as reminders of life outside of doctor's appointments and therapies. Having friends can be beneficial to mental health since they can provide amusement, spontaneity, and even diversion.

A special sense of companionship is provided by support groups that are started by friends or other cancer survivors. People can exchange experiences and tales here, creating a sense of community that is frequently lacking in conventional medical settings. These groups provide a judgment-free environment for patients to talk about the highs and lows of their journey. It can be comforting to hear others describe comparable difficulties and to realize that one is not fighting this battle alone.

The emotional toll on caregivers, whether they be friends or relatives, can be significant. They frequently have to balance taking care of themselves with helping someone they care about. It takes a great deal of emotional intelligence to navigate the variety of feelings that a caregiver may experience, which includes anxiety, despair, and frustration. Because caregivers' well-being has a direct impact on the standard of care they can deliver, self-care becomes crucial. It's critical that friends and family support them in taking breaks, engaging in hobbies, and expressing their own feelings.

In these interactions, open communication is essential. Families and friends should foster an environment where people can express their emotions without worrying about being judged. "How are you feeling today?" is a straightforward inquiry that can lead to more in-depth discussions. It enables caregivers to communicate their own difficulties and patients to disclose their vulnerabilities. This relationship strengthens support for one another and promotes a better comprehension of one another's backgrounds.

Maintaining relationships can be aided by technology, particularly when loved ones are separated by distance. Social networking, text messaging, and video chats offer channels for support that cut across regional borders. Receiving a video call from family or a text from a friend might provide someone going through treatment an instant emotional lift. No matter how far away they may be from their loved ones, patients are reminded that they are not alone by the simple act of reaching out.

Friends' and family's roles may change as patients move through their treatment process. First, there can be a surge of help, with family members willing to lend a hand. But as time goes on, the level of that support may change, which might occasionally make the patient feel alone. Even when the immediate crisis appears to have passed, it is crucial that friends and family stay informed about these changes and continue to provide support. Even when therapy is continuing or coming to an end, routine check-ins can help keep relationships strong and reaffirm that the patient is still loved and supported.

Another action that promotes hope is planning for the future. Talking about post-treatment objectives like vacation, new interests, or significant life events might help turn attention from the difficulties of treatment to the opportunities that lie ahead. This optimistic outlook can be inspiring because it serves as a reminder to all parties concerned that cancer is not the end of the world. Because they might offer resources or suggestions to help accomplish these objectives, loved ones can also participate meaningfully in these conversations.

The support network can be strengthened even more by exchanging resources and expertise. Friends and family can educate themselves on breast cancer, available treatments, and techniques for providing emotional support. Their comprehension allows them to provide more significant support. They can provide useful resources, such as books, podcasts, or neighborhood support groups, giving the patient and themselves information that could make the trip easier.

Families and friends may feel more purposeful if they take part in awareness-raising activities or fund-raising for breast cancer research. Engaging in such activities can bring loved ones together and channel their combined energy into action. Engaging in activities such as organizing a fundraiser, going for a walk, or even posting information on social media can be effective ways to show support and unity.

The experience of coping with breast cancer is ultimately shaped by the presence of family, friends, and caregivers. It is impossible to overestimate their capacity to offer social, emotional, and physical support. Resilience and hope, which are crucial components of the process of diagnosis, treatment, and recovery, are fostered by creating an atmosphere full of compassion, love, and proactive involvement. Relationships formed at this period can have a lasting impact on each person as they face their own obstacles, altering their perspective on both the illness and the deep bonds that get them through the most trying times.

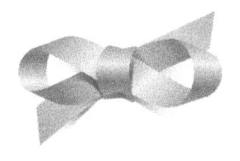

Getting in Touch with Survivor Communities

These areas, which are frequently full of common experiences and understanding, foster a community where people can get support and comfort from others who have gone through similar things. The experience of dealing with breast cancer can be lonely, but survivor communities provide a forum for empowerment, empathy, and connection.

These communities can take many different forms, which is one of their most alluring features. Survivors can connect through local support networks, social media groups, and online forums. Every platform has distinct qualities that meet a range of requirements. For people who might not yet feel comfortable talking about their experiences in public, online forums can be especially alluring since they provide anonymity. Without the stress of in-person interactions, survivors can ask questions, share personal tales, and exchange information here.

Conversely, social networking sites frequently provide a feeling of accessibility and immediacy. Survivors can interact with people across geographic boundaries by sharing their experiences and views with a wide audience. For instance, Facebook and Instagram have evolved into online galleries where users share their experiences via images, descriptions, and hashtags, demythologizing what it's like to live with breast cancer. These forums can emphasize persistence in the face of hardship by showcasing commonplace facts and victories.

The dynamic offered by local support groups is different. They offer a private space where people can get together, talk about their experiences, and develop bonds that go beyond the group gatherings. Face-to-face communication can be extremely healing, enabling survivors to connect emotionally in ways that are frequently more difficult to achieve online. Deeper discussions about anxieties, aspirations, and coping strategies can be facilitated by this personal touch, which can strengthen emotions of support and belonging.

Every relationship made in these communities has great power. Survivors frequently talk about the solace that comes from knowing that they are not alone in their difficulties. Sharing personal stories may validate thoughts and experiences, whether the topic is managing relationships, the mental toll of a diagnosis, or the physical changes brought on by therapy. For people who might experience isolation or misunderstanding in their day-to-day lives, this assurance is essential.

Additionally, survivor communities function as forums for advocacy and education. Many members of these forums act as unofficial teachers, imparting information on therapies, adverse effects, and services for recently diagnosed persons. By exchanging knowledge, survivors are empowered to take charge of their own health journeys and develop a sense of agency. These relationships frequently give rise to awareness efforts that raise awareness of the consequences of breast cancer and the significance of routine checkups.

Additionally, artistic expression frequently enters survivor communities. Writing, painting, or performing are examples of creative outlets that enable people to meaningfully digest their experiences. Sharing their artwork may be a potent storytelling tool for many survivors, helping them to connect their experiences with those of others. By enabling people to communicate feelings that might otherwise be difficult to articulate, creative expression can be a therapeutic tool.

Some people's involvement in these groups develops into a dedication to helping others, going beyond simple personal healing. In these groups, mentoring frequently occurs as survivors who have already made the journey share their knowledge with those who are just starting. Peer support like this can be extremely helpful in giving newly diagnosed people hope and practical coping mechanisms. It promotes a sense of resilience and togetherness by highlighting the continuation of the survivor experience.

Additionally, events like races, walks, and fundraisers are regularly held by survivor communities. In addition to increasing awareness and funding for breast cancer research, these events give survivors a chance to connect, exchange stories, and commemorate their experiences. Members' shared purpose can be strengthened by the positive and energizing energy of group participation. These events frequently provide people a sense of empowerment by serving as a reminder of the power that comes from being involved in the community.

Participating in these groups can also help to promote conversations about wellbeing and mental health. Following a breast cancer diagnosis, survivors frequently experience anxiety, despair, and other emotional difficulties. Communities dispel stigma and encourage people to get help when they need it by having candid conversations about these subjects. Professionals in the mental health field frequently take part in these forums, providing tools and coping mechanisms for the psychological effects of cancer. This kind of cooperation highlights the value of providing treatment that is holistic, taking into account both the journey's emotional and physical components.

Survivors frequently find a common language that goes beyond the details of their unique experiences as they bond with one another. This knowledge fosters an empathetic society in which people may help one another without passing judgment. Survivor communities typically place a high value on the act of listening since it may be incredibly therapeutic. By doing this, they provide a vulnerability-safe environment where people may communicate their worries and anxieties without worrying about being stigmatized.

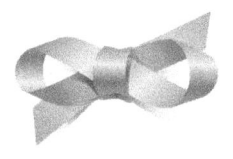

Locating Expert Assistance (Social Workers, Counselors)

THE EXPERIENCE OF DEALING with breast cancer is intense, frequently difficult, and fraught with psychological and emotional complications. It is impossible to overestimate the value of expert assistance during medical procedures and physical difficulties. Social workers and counselors are essential in offering the resources and emotional support required to go through this challenging journey.

Counselors are prepared with methods and resources to assist people in processing their emotions, anxieties, and doubts. Patients can share their feelings in a safe, judgment-free environment when they participate in therapy. Anxiety, despair, or a feeling of loneliness are common among people receiving treatment. People can better comprehend their emotional landscape by exploring these feelings with the assistance of a counselor. Healthy coping strategies are frequently the result of this knowledge, and they can be extremely helpful when stress levels are high.

Empowerment might come from the therapeutic alliance formed with a counselor. People can take back control of their story when they write about their experiences, changing from a passive to an active position in their journey. In order to help patients focus on their strengths and develop a healing mentality, counselors can also teach them techniques that foster emotional resilience. This method can be particularly helpful when dealing with the unknowns surrounding diagnosis and therapy. Through the development of an emotional management framework, patients might discover that their vulnerability is a strength.

Conversely, social workers provide an alternative but no less significant kind of assistance. They frequently specialize in helping people find services and navigating the healthcare system. It might be intimidating to deal with the intricacy of insurance procedures, treatment alternatives, and support services. Social workers can help people navigate these systems so they can get the community services and medical care they need. They are skilled at handling pragmatic issues like support groups, transportation services, and financial aid programs.

Social workers are adept at standing up for patients' rights in addition to providing logistical support. They can assist in removing obstacles to care, navigating any discrimination patients may encounter, and ensuring that they receive fair treatment. For members of underrepresented populations, who can face additional obstacles in obtaining care, this campaigning is especially crucial. By putting people in touch with helpful resources, social workers can help them feel less alone by fostering a sense of belonging and community.

Both social workers and counselors provide support groups in group settings where people can exchange stories and gain knowledge from one another. These get-togethers have the power to change people and foster a sense of unity among attendees. An atmosphere where people feel understood and validated is created through sharing tales. People are reminded that they are not alone in their challenges, which frequently lessens feelings of loneliness. The knowledge acquired from common experiences can have a profound effect, offering perceptions and coping mechanisms that others can relate to.

Counselors may use a variety of therapeutic methods that are suited to each client's needs in addition to conventional one-on-one treatment. Emotional well-being can be improved by methods including expressive arts therapy, mindfulness exercises, and cognitive-behavioral therapy (CBT). While mindfulness exercises promote stress reduction and present-moment awareness, cognitive behavioral therapy (CBT) can assist people in recognizing and combating harmful thought patterns. Counselors can encourage a comprehensive approach to rehabilitation by including various approaches into treatment.

Social workers frequently adopt a more community-focused strategy, concentrating on structural problems that affect people with breast cancer. They might try to find service gaps or push for legislative reforms that would give all patients better access to care. They can help create a more sympathetic and understanding healthcare environment by teaching medical professionals about the particular difficulties faced by patients with breast cancer. Patient opinions are heard and taken into account during decision-making thanks to this advocacy work.

Navigating the complexity of breast cancer requires people to get the correct professional support. Even if the path may seem overwhelming, getting help from social workers and counselors can reveal strategies to become resilient and heal. Their combined knowledge builds a network of support that not only attends to emotional needs but also gives people the tools they need to take control of their health and wellbeing.

When patients are thinking about their alternatives for help, it's critical that they contact with their social worker or counselor. For therapy to be effective, rapport and trust are essential. It should be easy for patients to voice their concerns and ask inquiries. A solid therapeutic connection can improve the whole experience by creating a healing and growth-promoting atmosphere.

Getting in touch with expert support can be a lifesaver in a world that can occasionally feel lonely. Social workers' and counselors' knowledge offers priceless resources outside of the professional context. These experts assist people in developing resilience, overcoming the challenges associated with their diagnosis, and finding strength they may not have known they had.

The presence of caring support can have a big impact as the trip progresses. Counselors and social workers enhance the experience of those dealing with breast cancer, whether through individual therapy, group sessions, or community resources. Through their advocacy, support, and insights, a more empowered approach to health and well-being is made possible, opening doors for resilience and hope even in the face of adversity.

Chapter 3

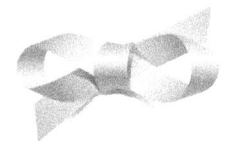

Examining Available Treatments

The type of breast cancer, its stage, the patient's medical history, and personal preferences are just a few of the many options available to them. For patients and their support networks to make well-informed decisions catered to their particular situation, they must have a thorough understanding of the various treatments.

One of the mainstays of treatment for breast cancer is frequently surgery. Mastectomy and lumpectomy are the two main surgical procedures. The goal of a lumpectomy is to preserve as much of the breast as possible by removing the tumor along with a tiny margin of surrounding tissue. Those who want to preserve the appearance of their breasts may find this choice especially alluring. However, depending on the extent of the cancer, a mastectomy entails removing either one or both breasts. Some people make this decision in order to lower their chance of recurrence, particularly when the tumor is aggressive or there is a significant family history of breast cancer.

Many people think about adjuvant therapy after surgery to reduce the likelihood of cancer recurring. After a lumpectomy, radiation therapy is frequently advised to eradicate any cancer cells that may still be present in the breast region. This treatment, which calls for several sessions spread over several weeks, uses high-energy rays directed at the afflicted area. For patients getting ready for this phase of their journey, it is essential to comprehend how radiation affects daily life, including possible side effects including weariness and skin irritation.

Another important therapeutic option is chemotherapy, especially for patients with aggressive breast cancer. Strong medications are used in this systemic therapy to eradicate cancer cells all across the body. Neoadjuvant therapy is the use of chemotherapy before to surgery to reduce tumor size and facilitate their removal. As an alternative, it might be administered to eradicate any remaining cancer cells following surgery. During therapy, patients should talk about any side effects that could affect their quality of life, such as nausea, hair loss, and changes in appetite.

Patients with hormone receptor-positive breast cancers, whose development is regulated by progesterone and estrogen, may benefit from hormonal therapy. By inhibiting these hormones or reducing their levels in the body, medications like aromatase inhibitors or tamoxifen can dramatically minimize the chance of recurrence. Patients and healthcare professionals must communicate often during this treatment, which is frequently taken for several years, in order to track side effects and general health.

In the battle against breast cancer, targeted medicines have become a ray of hope, especially for patients with HER2-positive tumors, which have a tendency to grow more quickly and aggressively. Trastuzumab (Herceptin) is one medication that targets the HER2 protein selectively, slowing or stopping the growth of cancer. These treatments frequently complement chemotherapy, increasing the treatment's overall efficacy. Patients should be made aware of the possibility of cardiac side effects from certain targeted treatments, which call for routine heart health monitoring.

Immunotherapy is becoming more popular as a treatment for some forms of breast cancer, especially triple-negative breast cancer, which is resistant to HER2-targeted or hormonal therapies. This novel method uses the body's immune system to identify and combat cancerous cells. As a result of a shift toward more individualized treatment paradigms, medications such as pembrolizumab (Keytruda) may be used in conjunction with chemotherapy for patients with advanced disease.

In the context of treatment, integrative methods are equally essential. Complementary therapies including yoga, acupuncture, and nutritional counseling can help patients cope with the negative effects of traditional treatments while also improving their general well-being. By creating connections with people who have gone through similar things, emotional assistance via counseling or support groups can offer priceless resources. Having a solid support system makes the trip less lonely for patients as they deal with the difficulties of treatment.

Throughout the course of treatment, patient education is still crucial. New treatments and clinical trials are made available as science advances, giving hope for improved results. Talking with medical professionals about these choices guarantees that people stay informed and in control. In order to promote a sense of agency during a period that may feel disempowering, each person's treatment plan should be tailored to their values, preferences, and lifestyle.

Additionally, healthcare professionals are essential in helping patients navigate this challenging environment. Questions and concerns can be handled in a collaborative relationship that is fostered by open communication. In order to enable patients to make well-informed decisions that align with their individual objectives, providers should take the time to thoroughly explain the reasoning behind each treatment option, including any potential risks and advantages.

It's critical for patients to accept the fact that choosing a course of treatment is not a straight line when they start this journey. Flexibility and adaptation are necessary as experiences and tastes change. Frequent follow-ups with medical professionals provide the chance to review the effectiveness of treatment and make any necessary modifications. Discussions regarding lifestyle decisions, physical health, and mental health support a holistic approach to care by bringing treatment into line with each patient's requirements and values.

Beyond therapy, awareness of breast cancer includes knowledge of the disease's wider effects on relationships and daily life. Raising community awareness creates support networks that have a big influence on patient experiences. Programs that encourage early detection through education and screening can result in better results and higher survival rates.

Resilience and the quest for knowledge are hallmarks of the path for those who get a breast cancer diagnosis. Patients who investigate treatment alternatives in a nurturing setting are more equipped to face their challenges with courage, optimism, and a more profound comprehension of their options. Every choice made along the way adds to a larger story of courage and recovery, highlighting the challenging but worthwhile process of overcoming breast cancer.

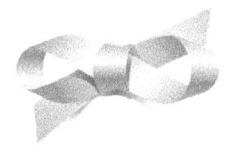

Surgery: Reconstructive Options, Mastectomy, and Lumpectomy

For patients with breast cancer, the two main surgical options are mastectomy and lumpectomy. Each has unique ramifications, benefits, and difficulties that impact a patient's journey on both a physical and emotional level.

A lumpectomy, sometimes referred to as breast-conserving surgery, attempts to preserve as much of the breast as possible while excising the tumor and a tiny margin of surrounding tissue. Because it can limit bodily changes while yet managing the malignancy, this technique has received a lot of support. The desire to preserve their breasts is a strong argument for many people to get a lumpectomy. Furthermore, research suggests that for some forms of breast cancer, radiation therapy after a lumpectomy may be just as successful as mastectomy.

Nevertheless, this choice is rarely simple. The suitability of a lumpectomy depends on the tumor's form, size, and stage as well as individual preferences and genetic considerations. Patients may struggle with the emotional burden of their decision, balancing their fear of a cancer return against their wish to preserve their body image. During this stage, discussions with medical professionals are crucial because they provide insight into the prognosis and the need for additional treatments, such radiation, which usually comes after a lumpectomy.

A mastectomy, on the other hand, entails the removal of the entire breast along with any surrounding lymph nodes. For people with advanced cancers or those with a strong family history, this operation may seem more drastic, but it frequently gives them a feeling of closure. Some patients believe that a mastectomy provides a more thorough method of cancer removal, especially in cases where the tumor is big or multifocal.

Mastectomy might have a significant emotional aftereffect. As they deal with changes to their bodies and identities, many patients feel bereaved or grieved. At this point, discussing reconstructive possibilities becomes crucial. Following a mastectomy, reconstructive surgery can aid in regaining confidence and a sense of normalcy. Autologous tissue reconstruction, which uses tissue from other regions of the body, and implant-based reconstruction are two options available to patients.

Reconstruction based on implants is frequently the simpler choice. It usually entails putting a silicone or saline implant behind the chest muscle, which may be done right once following a mastectomy or later. This approach is attractive since it requires less significant surgery and has a comparatively short recovery period. It does, however, have a number of drawbacks, such as the possibility of infection, scarring, and the requirement for additional procedures to replace the implants.

Conversely, autologous tissue reconstruction uses the patient's own tissue to form a new breast shape, as in the TRAM flap or DIEP flap operations. Because it uses the body's natural substance, this method can offer a more natural appearance and feel. Nevertheless, it frequently necessitates a more involved surgical process, longer recuperation periods, and possible effects on the donor site, such weakening in the abdomen or altered sensation.

Reconstruction is a very personal choice that can be impacted by a number of variables, such as lifestyle, general health, and body image. During this phase, it can be quite helpful to have the support of peers who have been through similar experiences, family, and medical experts. Speaking with someone who has had the same operation can be enlightening and consoling for many people.

During this process, decision-making heavily relies on awareness and knowledge. Patients can make educated selections if they are aware of the specifics of each surgical procedure, the possible risks and advantages, and the available reconstructive options. Patient advocacy groups frequently connect people with others who have experienced similar difficulties and provide information. In addition to providing emotional support and useful guidance, these networks can help people feel more connected to one another during this difficult time.

In addition, improvements in technology and surgical methods have helped individuals with breast cancer achieve better results. One less invasive method to screen for cancer spread is sentinel node biopsy, which has become commonplace. By reducing the need for significant lymph node resection, this invention improves recovery and minimizes problems.

Medical experts' approaches to therapy are also changing as a result of new studies on the psychological effects of breast cancer surgery. Many hospitals now include counseling services, support groups, and educational workshops in their care models because they recognize that mental health is just as important as physical healing. In order to address the sometimes disregarded mental health component of their journey, patients are urged to talk about their concerns regarding surgery, body image, and the future.

Being proactive can have a big impact on the experience of those dealing with the effects of breast cancer. Patients can be empowered by keeping lines of communication open with medical teams regarding surgical alternatives, anticipated results, and personal feelings. Every stage, from diagnosis to therapy, gives them a chance to participate in their care, making them feel informed and supported.

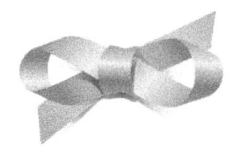

Radiation and Chemotherapy: What to Expect

Chemotherapy targets and destroys rapidly dividing cancer cells by using potent medications. This systemic treatment can target tiny cells that may have spread throughout the body in addition to obvious malignancies. Chemotherapy regimens are usually given in cycles and are tailored to the patient's characteristics, cancer type, and stage. Since chemotherapy can present a number of mental and physical difficulties, many people may find their first experience with it to be overwhelming.

Chemotherapy patients frequently describe a variety of side effects. Vomiting and nausea are common, but they can be lessened by a number of drugs. As a result of the body exerting itself to counteract the effects of the medications and the illness itself, fatigue frequently also develops. Another well-known adverse effect is hair loss; many people have thinning or total hair loss, which can have a big impact on their self-esteem. Some people find solace in support groups, where they can exchange stories and coping mechanisms.

Additionally, chemotherapy may affect the immune system, increasing a patient's vulnerability to infections. Frequent blood tests aid in tracking these developments and assist medical professionals modify treatment regimens to protect patients. Nutrition and food are important during this time since a balanced diet can help you stay strong and have energy. Equally important, hydration can improve general health and reduce weariness.

Radiation therapy, on the other hand, is a localized treatment intended to target particular regions where cancer cells are found. It usually comes after surgery, particularly if there is a chance that the tumor excision will leave cancer behind. Eliminating any cancer cells that remain and lowering the chance of recurrence are the objectives. In order to minimize exposure to nearby healthy tissues, this treatment uses high-energy photons that are similar to X-rays and are carefully delivered to the afflicted area.

To ensure accuracy, sophisticated imaging techniques are used to map the precise treatment region during the radiation planning phase. The actual therapy sessions are typically short, lasting only a few minutes at most. Most patients receive treatment five days a week for several weeks, though the number of sessions can vary.

Although they frequently differ from those linked to chemotherapy, adverse effects are also possible with radiation. Redness, peeling, or sensitivity in the treated area are common symptoms of skin irritation. Persistent fatigue might show up as a general feeling of exhaustion that might not go away with rest. Radiation exposure over time can alter the skin or underlying tissues, occasionally resulting in scarring or fibrosis.

Radiation and chemotherapy can also cause emotional reactions. Anxiety may result from the ambiguity about the effectiveness of treatment. By demythologizing treatment procedures, conversations with medical teams can provide patients a better understanding of what to anticipate. Participating in social networks, such as community activities, support groups, or counseling, can offer vital emotional outlets.

Communication is still essential during the course of treatment. Concerns regarding side effects, progress, and necessary treatment plan modifications can be addressed by maintaining an open line of communication with medical professionals. Understanding their treatment frequently empowers patients, giving them a sense of agency throughout their journey. Talking about how it affects day-to-day activities like employment, social connections, and family dynamics is also crucial. Patients can use these discussions to help them make well-informed decisions that suit their preferences and values.

During therapy, preserving a sense of normalcy can greatly improve quality of life. In order to manage their stress and discomfort, many patients look into complementary therapies like yoga, acupuncture, or mindfulness exercises. Every person has a different journey, therefore what suits one person might not suit another. Finding what promotes comfort and resilience can be accomplished by trying out different approaches.

Throughout the course of treatment, nutrition is still essential. Aversions to particular foods may develop in some patients, or their tastes may shift. It can be helpful to maintain a flexible diet plan that emphasizes nutrient-dense, enticing meals. Speaking with nutritionists can help ensure that the body gets the right fuel for healing and resiliency during treatment by offering customized guidance to address particular needs.

Although receiving treatment for breast cancer might occasionally feel lonely, many people find comfort in their shared experiences. Making connections with people who have experienced similar things can provide solace, friendship, and comprehension. These relationships, whether made through official support groups or unofficial get-togethers, can cultivate hope and a feeling of belonging.

Many patients report changes in perspective as their treatment goes on, which frequently results in a greater appreciation for life's little pleasures. This life-changing experience could inspire introspection and make people think about what really important to them.

Taking an intentional approach to every day can act as a compass. Enjoying joyful pursuits, such as hobbies, time spent with loved ones, or just taking in the scenery, can offer much-needed respite from the demands of medical care. Every action, whether a minor triumph or a major turning point, can strengthen the inner strength.

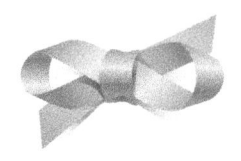

Complementary and Alternative Medicines

EVERY PERSON LOOKS for strategies to empower oneself in the face of uncertainty as they navigate the complicated and emotionally taxing road that is breast cancer. In addition to traditional medical treatments, alternative and complementary therapies have become important options for many people. These treatments provide a comprehensive approach, addressing the emotional, psychological, and spiritual facets of the illness in addition to its physical manifestations, which frequently coexist with a cancer diagnosis.

Practices that can be distinguished from conventional medicine are included in alternative therapies. These consist of methods like herbal medicine, acupuncture, and nutritional supplements. Many people report improvements in their general well-being, even though the scientific community frequently questions these techniques for their empirical backing. For example, acupuncture has been investigated for its ability to reduce chemotherapy-related discomfort, nausea, and exhaustion. Thin needles are inserted into particular body spots in an effort to promote healing and restore equilibrium. Some people find that the act itself turns into a self-care ritual, reaffirming their sense of agency in the face of helplessness.

Another option is herbal medicine, which has a long history and is used in many different cultures. While some herbs, like ashwagandha, may help control stress and anxiety, others, like turmeric and ginger, are known for their anti-inflammatory qualities. Herbal supplements must be used carefully because they may interact dangerously with prescription drugs. Working together with medical professionals to make these decisions can maximize the positive effects and reduce any potential negative ones.

Conversely, complementary therapies are meant to supplement traditional treatments rather than take their place. Breast cancer patients are increasingly using practices including yoga, mindfulness meditation, and guided visualization. Yoga has been linked to increases in physical stamina, mental resilience, and quality of life because of its combination of physical postures and breath control. Regular practice may help people develop a sense of calm despite the stress of therapy by lowering anxiety and exhaustion, according to research.

The psychological advantages of mindfulness meditation, which emphasizes present-moment awareness without passing judgment, have also been emphasized. When dealing with the stress of cancer, this practice can help people manage their emotions, reduce depressive symptoms, and improve their general wellbeing. Visualizing peaceful environments or successful outcomes is known as guided imagery, and it can be a very effective technique for pain management and relaxation. By providing mental anchors, these strategies help people stay rooted in the here and now rather than letting their thoughts wander into future-focused concern.

The course of breast cancer is significantly influenced by nutrition. A plant-based diet high in fruits, vegetables, whole grains, and healthy fats is frequently emphasized in complementary dietary therapy. Certain food choices may improve immune function and even aid the body's reaction to therapy, according to some research. For example, diets high in antioxidants may help reduce oxidative stress brought on by cancer and its treatments. Nonetheless, the field of diet in cancer treatment is complicated, with different guidelines depending on the specific situation. Consulting with an oncology-focused registered dietician can offer tailored advice and promote long-lasting improvements.

Several complementary therapies meet the need for emotional support, which is essential to handling the experience of breast cancer. Creative methods for expressing emotions that might be hard to put into words are provided by music therapy and art therapy. These therapies promote healing and connection by enabling people to use creativity to process their experiences. While music can arouse feelings and memories and offer solace during trying times, expressive art can act as a cathartic outlet.

Online or in-person support groups are now crucial for helping breast cancer patients connect and build a sense of community. It is possible to reduce feelings of loneliness and foster a sense of belonging by exchanging experiences with those going through comparable difficulties. Hearing about others' tenacity, optimism, and survival gives many people courage and fosters a sense of empowerment among all.

Furthermore, incorporating bodywork therapies like massage or reflexology into one's self-care routine can ease physical discomfort and encourage relaxation. Massage has been shown to lower anxiety, boost general quality of life, and improve sleep quality. It is said that reflexology, which entails applying pressure to particular areas on the hands or feet, encourages balance and relaxation throughout the body. In addition to treating physical discomfort, these therapies promote a stronger mind-body bond and a greater understanding of one's own needs.

Navigating the path of breast cancer may also be significantly influenced by spirituality. Investigating spiritual activities can offer solace and purpose to some people during turbulent times. This investigation could involve prayer, meditation, or spending time in nature. People can discover serenity and understanding by interacting with their spirituality, which also helps them make sense of their experiences and find hope when things get tough.

Even though investigating complementary and alternative therapies can be very helpful, people must continue to be informed and involved in their treatment choices. It's critical to keep lines of communication open with medical professionals regarding any therapies that are selected. A coordinated approach to care is ensured by this partnership, reducing risks and optimizing advantages. It is crucial to understand that no one strategy is always successful and that what suits one individual might not suit another.

Alternative and complementary therapies can be effective allies for people navigating their own experiences with breast cancer. They give people the chance to regain control over their health and well-being by offering chances for empowerment, self-discovery, and healing. These methods, which include acupuncture, mindfulness, diet, and artistic expression, provide a variety of routes to strength and resilience. Adopting this multidimensional strategy respects the interwoven strands of physical, emotional, and spiritual well-being that characterize the journey through breast cancer and recognizes the complexity of the human experience.

Chapter 4

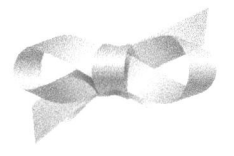

Managing the Emotional Rollercoaster

Managing the emotional terrain following a breast cancer diagnosis is similar to navigating a complex tapestry made of strands of fear, uncertainty, and fortitude. People struggle with the significant effects of their diagnosis on themselves and their loved ones at every point of this journey, which necessitates a delicate balancing act. The complexities of the emotional rollercoaster are revealed in this investigation, illustrating the various ways in which people might experience and react to this momentous occasion.

Following the diagnosis, a range of emotions may surface, frequently starting with shock. The news's starkness might make people feel as though time has stopped for a second, leaving them stunned. Anxiety often arises when the reality sets in, causing questions to whirl like a raging storm. How will this affect my future? What impact will this have on my family? Can I handle the challenges that lie ahead? These ideas frequently consume the mind, resulting in an unending cycle from which it can be challenging to break free.

Understanding that the emotional turmoil is shared as well as personal is crucial during this early stage. These emotions are frequently mirrored by friends and family, who also have their own worries. The general anxiety might intensify feelings, resulting in a tense environment where powerlessness and fear rule. It becomes crucial to have open channels of communication in order to create a space where emotions can be aired and accepted. By turning loneliness into a shared experience, this support system helps lessen the load.

The emotional terrain changes once more as the medical process progresses, including consultations, examinations, and treatment options conversations. Many people struggle with their dread of the unknown while navigating the complexities of medical jargon, leaving them in a condition of limbo. Long wait times between consultations are common, and they are frequently accompanied by an increased sense of vulnerability. It's normal to feel as though you're walking a tightrope between hope and despair. In the midst of the chaos, maintaining a sense of regularity through daily rituals might allow for little periods of relaxation.

But in the midst of the chaos, hope is a strong force that can appear suddenly. Finding little triumphs can lift your spirits, whether they come from encouraging words from loved ones, positive news from a medical professional, or even significant life events. Some people find that experimenting with creative outlets, such as journaling, painting, or music, provides a cathartic release and a healthy way to express their feelings. Clarity can be gained by producing, which turns suffering into something concrete and significant.

The emotional rollercoaster may get more intense during treatment. Physical difficulties brought on by radiation, chemotherapy, or surgery might exacerbate mental problems. Feelings of loss or inadequacy might result from physical discomfort, changes in appearance, and fatigue. Instead of repressing these feelings, it is imperative to face them. Online or in-person support groups can provide as a safe haven for exchanging stories and coping mechanisms, reaffirming that one is not traveling this path alone.

During this time, emotional highs and lows become a natural part of existence. While some days could seem like a journey toward hope, others might feel like a descent into gloom. It is essential to let oneself feel the whole range of emotions because doing so can help one better grasp how resilient they are. Whether via mindfulness, meditation, or just letting oneself rest, practicing self-compassion during these trying times can set the groundwork for both physical and emotional healing.

A change in viewpoint frequently happens as treatment goes on. Many people say they have a renewed appreciation for the small things in life, including spending time with loved ones, taking nature walks, or having quiet times to think. In times of turbulence, this thankfulness can act as a strong anchor and provide stability. Realizing that life is a gift, despite its unpredictable nature, can give each day purpose and emphasize the need of living completely in the moment.

But the path to recovery might be paved with obstacles that go beyond the short-term health issues. Survivorship frequently entails a unique set of emotional challenges, such as identity changes, reevaluating life goals, and concern about recurrence. As people struggle with the before and after of their experiences, a sense of loss may accompany the change. Processing these complicated emotions can be facilitated by participating in supportive therapies, such as art therapy, counseling, or physical exercise.

As one travels this path, developing resilience emerges as a key topic. Resilience includes growth and adaptation in the face of hardship, not just getting back up after a setback. Every person's journey is different, influenced by their coping strategies, support networks, and past experiences. Feelings of powerlessness can be changed into a sense of agency by accepting the story of one's own experience.

Another important factor in this process is awareness. Feelings of powerlessness can be lessened by educating oneself about breast cancer, including its dangers, available treatments, and support systems. People are empowered by knowledge and can take an active role in their own healing and treatment. By exchanging experiences and learning from others, advocacy organizations may foster a strong sense of belonging and community, which can further strengthen this sense of agency.

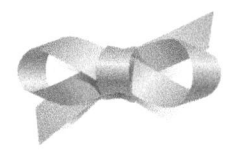

Controlling Anxiety and Fear

Throughout a breast cancer journey, fear and worry can be overwhelming and impact all facets of life. Relationships, health, and general well-being are all impacted by these strong emotions, which frequently overflow into daily activities. Navigating the road to recovery, however, requires recognizing and dealing with these emotions. Comprehending the subtleties of anxiety and dread associated with breast cancer can result in practical methods for handling them, enabling people to proceed with courage and optimism.

A diagnosis of breast cancer can kick off a chain reaction of emotions. Questions concerning mortality, available treatments, and the effect on loved ones frequently follow the first shock. There may be particular anxieties at each stage: diagnosis, therapy, and after treatment. Some people can become paralyzed by their fear of the unknown. What will be the course of treatment? How will it impact day-to-day living? What happens if the cancer comes back? These inquiries may cause mental haze, which makes it difficult to concentrate on the here and now.

Anxiety can take many different forms. Physical symptoms such an elevated heart rate, trouble sleeping, or stomach problems may be experienced by certain people. Others may become enmeshed in an unrelenting pattern of pessimistic ideas. It's critical to recognize these responses. They are a normal reaction to an overwhelming circumstance rather than an indication of weakness.

A potent tool in the fight against anxiety and terror is awareness. By practicing mindfulness, people can stop the cycle of worry and re-establish a connection with the present. One can become grounded in the present moment by practicing methods like yoga, meditation, and deep breathing. These exercises promote the nonjudgmental, peaceful observation of feelings and thoughts. By practicing mindfulness, one can become more adept at navigating the emotional turbulence and create quiet moments in the middle of chaos.

Creating a network of support can also be quite helpful. Building relationships with people who have gone through comparable experiences promotes empathy and comradery. Online or in-person support groups can provide a secure environment for discussing successes and anxieties. People can take comfort in shared experiences in these settings, realizing they are not alone in their difficulties.

Speaking with medical professionals can assist to clarify the path forward. Lack of knowledge is frequently the root cause of fear. Open communication with physicians and nurses can help to define expectations for recovery, possible side effects, and treatment plans. People can feel less anxious and be more empowered to actively participate in their treatment if they know exactly what to expect. During doctor's appointments, keeping a notebook to record queries and worries can be a useful tool to make sure that nothing is overlooked.

Additionally, exercise is essential for anxiety management. Endorphins, the body's natural mood enhancers, are known to be released during exercise. Walking and dancing are two examples of activities that might divert attention from negative thoughts. They enhance general wellbeing and give a feeling of achievement. Establishing a routine that includes physical activity might help people regain some control over their lives during a period when many things feel uncertain by establishing a sense of normalcy.

Since nutrition is essential to mental health, it should not be disregarded. Mood and energy levels can be significantly impacted by eating a balanced diet. Brain health can be supported by foods high in vitamins, antioxidants, and omega-3 fatty acids. Emotional stability can also be achieved by minimizing sugar and caffeine intake and drinking plenty of water. Making meals, whether by yourself or with family, may make dining a loving activity that strengthens feelings of warmth and caring.

Another way to handle emotions is through artistic expression. People can convey emotions that may be hard to put into words via painting, writing, or playing music. Anxiety can be released through creative pursuits, which turn it into something material. In addition to boosting confidence during a period when self-doubt may surface, these activities can help cultivate a sense of accomplishment.

It is impossible to overestimate the significance of self-compassion. It's crucial to let oneself experience anxiety and terror guilt-free. One feels validated when they are told that it's acceptable to have a variety of emotions. Resilience can be developed by engaging in self-kindness practices, such as self-care routines, gentle reminders, or affirmations. Joyful pursuits, including hobbies or time spent in nature, might function as a buffer against the stress that comes with having cancer.

Fear can give way to appreciation when one is grateful. Perspectives might be reframed by keeping a gratitude diary in which one records daily or weekly moments of delight or thanks. By encouraging people to see the bright side of hardship, this approach builds resilience and optimism. Connecting with loved ones during these times helps deepen bonds and build a positive support system.

It's also critical to understand that dealing with worry and fear is a nonlinear process. It's quite common for some days to feel easier than others. Growth and comprehension are made possible by accepting the emotional landscape's ups and downs. A sense of success can be strengthened by acknowledging and celebrating minor accomplishments, such as finishing a treatment cycle, having a meaningful conversation, or just getting out of bed.

Getting expert assistance can be a beneficial part of the process. Counselors or therapists that specialize in cancer-related issues can provide coping mechanisms that are customized for each patient. For example, cognitive-behavioral therapy can assist in reframing negative thought patterns and substituting them with more positive narratives. These experts can help people find their footing in the face of uncertainty by offering advice on how to handle difficult emotions.

It can be consoling to keep in mind that anxiety and fear are normal human emotions as the journey progresses. There is no right or incorrect way to feel about breast cancer; everyone's journey is different. A deeper awareness of oneself and a greater appreciation for the trip ahead might result from embracing this complexity and applying useful techniques for regulating emotions. Marking off breast cancer is about living completely, with strength, hope, and a new sense of purpose, not just about surviving.

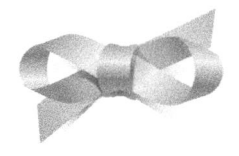

Adapting to Shifts in Body Image

A breast cancer diagnosis can cause significant and very personal changes to one's body image. Navigating a terrain full of physical, emotional, and psychological changes—each requiring a unique form of resilience—is a common part of the journey. Many people find that this journey involves more than simply bodily changes; it also involves reinventing their identity and sense of worth in the midst of hardship.

Surgery such a mastectomy or lumpectomy is often required to treat breast cancer, which can change the shape and look of the body. Feelings of vulnerability, loss, and grief may be triggered by these changes. The breasts are more than just bodily components; they are a component of one's identity and self-expression, frequently signifying femininity and sexuality. A crisis of confidence may result from the psychological effects of losing a breast or from changes in size or shape. Many people struggle with issues related to femininity, desirability, and their general self-perception.

Support networks are essential during this time. Although family, friends, and medical professionals can provide support and empathy, the experience is still very personal. Finding one's voice amid the clamor of viewpoints and well-intentioned counsel is crucial for people. While some people might find comfort in journaling or introspection, others might choose to express their emotions in public. Establishing a forum for emotional expression—whether via writing, painting, or dialogue—can be a potent release.

Real options that can help with the transition include wigs, prosthetics, and clothing made to be comfortable after surgery. Finding and donning these things might help people feel more normal. After a significant transformation, many discover that altering their look may be empowering and a means of reclaiming their identity. As people try out several styles that fit with their new self-image, this journey might inspire creativity.

Over the course of this journey, one's relationship with their body changes. Feelings of estrangement may arise at first from a strong focus on the obvious scars, changes in skin texture, or hair loss. But as time goes on, some people start to see their bodies as representations of strength and resiliency rather than just as beautiful objects. Whether it's yoga, walking, or dancing, physical activity can help one develop a stronger bond with their body. Instead of lamenting the body's changes, movement becomes a means to celebrate its abilities.

Body image and mental health are interwoven, especially when it comes to cancer. The physical changes may be accompanied by anxiety and sadness, which can exacerbate feelings of inadequacy. A secure environment for navigating these complicated emotions can be found by seeking professional assistance, such as therapy or counseling. Cognitive-behavioral methods can assist people in reframing negative body image ideas into more positive statements about their identity and self-worth.

Support groups are also very important. A sense of belonging can be developed by sharing experiences with those who are familiar with the trip. People can be motivated to accept their own changes by hearing tales of acceptance, resiliency, and hope. Realizing that one is not alone in one's challenges is frequently the key to the power of shared experiences.

Perceptions of body image can be greatly influenced by media representation. One's self-image can be strengthened or weakened by how breast cancer survivors are portrayed in the media and in advertisements. People must develop a personal story that is consistent with their reality and critically assess the messages they are given by outside sources. It can be encouraging and uplifting to find role models who represent a range of experiences.

Deep breathing exercises and meditation are examples of mindfulness techniques that can be used as coping mechanisms. By encouraging people to remain in the now, these techniques help them to accept their existing circumstances. Self-compassion can be fostered via mindfulness, enabling people to treat themselves with kindness throughout this trying period. More resilience and emotional balance can result from adopting mental health practices.

A lot of people find strength in advocacy or community involvement, which can transform their experience from one of victimization to empowerment. Sharing personal tales, taking part in fundraising events, and running awareness campaigns can all help people feel like they have a purpose. People may become more proud and feel more in control of their story as a result of this renewed emphasis.

Whether via formal religion or one's own convictions, spirituality can also be consoling. Many people find comfort in rituals that validate their identity and connection to something greater than themselves, and they find strength in their faith or spiritual activities. A framework for comprehending suffering, recovery, and personal development may be provided by this dimension.

Finally, the process of changing one's body image is not a straight line. It frequently entails failures, periods of uncertainty, and feelings of inadequacy that might reappear without warning. People might develop tolerance and self-compassion by accepting this ups and downs. Developing a toolkit of coping mechanisms, such as self-care routines and relationships with supportive people, can enable people to deal with life's emotional challenges in a resilient manner.

While dealing with breast cancer and its aftermath can be difficult, it can also be a time of significant change. A deeper awareness of oneself and fresh views can result from changes in body image, even though they can also cause pain. Accepting the journey with all of its ups and downs can help people develop and heal in unexpected ways by serving as a reminder of their resilience, optimism, and potential for rebirth.

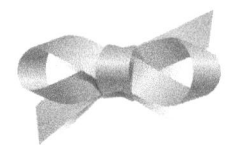

Developing Mindfulness and Resilience

RESILIENCE IS THE CAPACITY to adjust and flourish in the face of hardship; it goes beyond simple endurance. Building resilience for people with breast cancer entails cultivating an attitude that welcomes change and encourages emotional adaptability. Recognizing emotions like fear, grief, and rage as normal reactions to a diagnosis that changes one's life is the first step in this process. Instead of repressing these feelings, people can make room for them so they can really feel the intensity of what they are going through. A greater awareness of one's emotional terrain and a feeling of agency in the face of difficulties can result from this method.

Having social support is essential for developing resilience. Relationships with friends, family, and support groups can offer a feeling of acceptance and comprehension. Feelings of loneliness can be lessened by exchanging experiences with people who are traveling similar routes. These connections provide support and affirmation, creating a sense of unity that enables people to confront their challenges head-on. People frequently find comfort as well as useful coping and healing techniques through this sharing.

By bringing people back to the present, mindfulness as a practice enhances resilience. It promotes a sense of calm in the midst of chaos by promoting an awareness of ideas and feelings without passing judgment. A deeper awareness of the body and its sensations can be developed through mindfulness exercises including meditation, mindful walking, and deep breathing. This can be quite helpful to someone who is receiving treatment. Mindfulness promotes concentration on the present moment rather than dwelling on the past or worrying about the future. This change can improve emotional health, lessen stress, and lessen anxiety.

People can detach themselves from negative thought patterns by practicing mindfulness, which helps them observe their thoughts and feelings. For example, surges of worry and uncertainty are common during treatment. Mindfulness teaches the art of observation, which involves identifying ideas like "I'm scared" without necessarily believing them, as an alternative to being overcome by these feelings. This exercise helps people feel in control by reminding them that although they can't always control their situation, they can control how they react to it.

When dealing with the physical side effects of breast cancer treatment, resilience and mindfulness can be especially effective. Radiation or chemotherapy side effects may cause weariness and discomfort. In this situation, mindfulness can assist people in becoming more aware of their body and identifying feelings without passing judgment. Because of this understanding, they are able to react to their physical condition with empathy instead of annoyance. Rather than resisting weariness, they should welcome it as a signal to take a break and take care of themselves, developing a loving bond with their body at a period of significant transition.

Realistic goal-setting is another aspect of cultivating a resilient attitude. Small, attainable goals can give you direction and a sense of achievement. A sense of purpose can be created, for instance, by concentrating on everyday activities like going for a quick walk, engaging in mindfulness for a little while, or contacting a friend. Every goal accomplished, no matter how minor, strengthens the person's capacity for adaptation and coping. When these minor triumphs add up over time, they strengthen resilience, which serves as a basis for handling bigger obstacles.

Furthermore, incorporating artistic endeavors within the path helps improve awareness and resilience. People can process their feelings and experiences by using art, writing, or music as potent self-expression tools. The mind is frequently stimulated by creative pursuits in a way that promotes flow, a profound state of concentration and immersion. This interaction can offer relief from tension and worry, fostering a space for recovery and introspection. Being creative encourages people to be present and delve into their inner worlds, which is a sort of mindfulness in and of itself.

Another component of resilience, gratitude, has the power to change viewpoints under trying circumstances. Even modest acts of thankfulness can foster an appreciation for the happy times that occur in the middle of the hardship. The focus might be shifted from what is lost to what is left by keeping a gratitude diary in which one records everyday moments of thankfulness, such as a sunny day, a warm cup of tea, or encouraging friends. By emphasizing assets and characteristics that might otherwise go overlooked, this change not only promotes a more optimistic attitude but also strengthens resilience.

Seeking professional assistance can help improve resilience and mindfulness in addition to personal efforts. A secure environment for addressing anxieties, creating coping mechanisms, and exploring emotions can be found in therapy or counseling. Experts in mindfulness-based practices can lead people through methods specific to their own situation, promoting a better comprehension of how to develop resilience and present. Additionally, support groups provide the chance to interact with people who have gone through similar things, strengthening the bonds of camaraderie and solidarity.

In the end, dealing with breast cancer is a very unique and complex experience. Every person's journey is different, influenced by their feelings, experiences, and reactions to obstacles. People can embrace their experiences with a sense of agency and hope by practicing mindfulness and resilience. People can deal with the challenges of their diagnosis with a great sense of strength by cultivating emotional flexibility, accepting the present, and developing relationships with others. This will turn their experience into one of awareness and growth.

CHAPTER 5

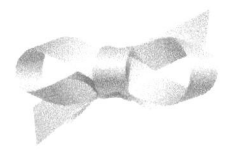

The Treatment's Aftereffects

The decisions taken during therapy and the tools available for rehabilitation can make this time as complicated as the diagnosis itself.

Many survivors experience a variety of physical side effects from procedures like radiation, chemotherapy, and surgery. Long after therapy is over, fatigue may persist as a recalcitrant reminder of the body's battle. Physical changes, such as changes in look and body image, can be a major obstacle for certain people. Feelings of loss or uncertainty might result from surgical scarring, changes in breast size or form, and other physical changes. The difficulty of balancing one's perception of oneself with the physical world becomes a recurring theme. It frequently takes time, patience, and support to embrace a new sense of self.

After treatment, survivors must navigate the psychological terrain, which can have significant emotional effects. Long after medical procedures stop, the experience of breast cancer can evoke a sense of vulnerability. Recurrence anxiety may be present in the background and take many different forms, such as restless nights, ongoing concern, or an excessive need for validation. Because of how exhausting this increased awareness may be, some people turn to counseling or support groups where they can discuss their experiences and find solace. People are frequently forced to face their fears and anxieties as a result of the emotional rollercoaster, which helps them better comprehend their own resilience.

Following treatment, social dynamics often change. Social circles may grow or shrink and relationships may change in response to the needs and experiences of the survivor. While some people may develop closer bonds with friends who provide constant support, others may find themselves estranged from friends who find it difficult to comprehend the intricacies of their path. As loved ones adjust to new circumstances, family responsibilities may also shift. Those in the immediate vicinity may be impacted by the survivor's experience. The true nature of connections and community can be revealed by navigating these changed dynamics, which can be both difficult and illuminating.

Many survivors find themselves reassessing their values and lifestyle choices as they think back on their experience. A reevaluation of what really matters is typically prompted by the experience, which frequently acts as a catalyst for change. As a way to take back control of their lives, some people could start eating better, exercising, and practicing mindfulness. This renewed dedication to self-care can take many different forms, such as regular exercise or pursuing creative endeavors that give one a feeling of direction. Many see these adjustments as a deliberate choice to respect their path and cultivate a revitalized feeling of wellbeing.

Following therapy, advocacy frequently assumes a central role. Many breast cancer survivors are driven to tell their story, spread awareness, and add to the larger conversation about the disease. Participation in community organizations, fundraising initiatives, and awareness campaigns can result from this desire to effect change. By taking on advocacy responsibilities, survivors elevate the voices of those who might not feel heard in addition to their own. By enabling people to turn their experiences into meaningful action, this participation can be a potent healing aid.

Another aspect of the post-treatment environment is navigating the healthcare system. Survivors frequently have to deal with continuing screenings, follow-up visits, and possible treatment side effects. This navigation can be intimidating, especially if they run into obstacles to care or conflicting medical advice. When survivors speak out for their own needs and desires, the value of having a supportive healthcare team becomes clear. Developing a rapport with healthcare professionals who are aware of their particular circumstances can empower survivors and enable them to actively participate in their recovery after treatment.

During this time, spirituality and introspection frequently gain prominence. Some people's experiences with cancer cause them to reevaluate their ideals and beliefs. Through personal rituals, organized religion, or a connection to nature, this reflection can result in a deeper spiritual connection. Journaling, yoga, meditation, and other mindfulness-promoting practices provide comfort to many. These exercises provide a technique to anchor oneself in the face of uncertainty in addition to providing relief from the erratic emotions.

Even in the midst of the upheaval, survivors frequently find themselves looking for a semblance of normalcy as they embark on this new chapter. Small daily routines, rekindling interests, or welcoming new experiences are some ways that this urge can show up. Establishing a schedule that includes enjoyable activities might serve as a much-needed anchor. Survivors frequently find happiness in the most mundane situations and rediscover significance in routines that previously seemed unimportant.

The idea of community becomes crucial when dealing with treatment's aftereffects. Whether through official groups or casual get-togethers, many survivors look for support systems that relate to their stories. These relationships provide a forum for exchanging tales, commemorating achievements, and providing support during trying times. As survivors discover they are not traveling alone, the power of group healing becomes evident, creating a sense of community that can be incredibly healing.

During this stage of life, resilience becomes a major focus. The process of removing breast cancer turns into a chance for personal development and transformation rather than only a survival adventure. Every action, whether it be in the direction of activism, recovery, or self-discovery, adds to a story of hope and strength. It's a complicated tapestry that depicts the many facets of recovery, woven from both triumphant and vulnerable moments.

Treatment for breast cancer has its own set of difficulties, but it also brings with it fresh opportunities and viewpoints. Survivors are more than just people who have survived a horrific event; they are active contributors to the ongoing discussion about community, wellbeing, and health. Although the path may be uncertain, there is a chance for significant change within that uncertainty.

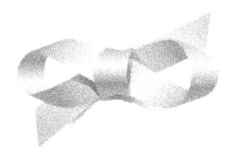

Honoring Achievements and Resilience

Significant events that signify not just the passage of time but also the development of strength, resiliency, and hope are known as milestones in the journey through breast cancer. Regardless of their size, these turning points act as checkpoints along a journey of change and uncertainty. They serve as a reminder to survivors that life can be rich and meaningful even in the face of adversity.

The diagnosis itself frequently marks the first significant turning point. Receiving that news can be a confusing time that sets off a chain reaction of emotions. A dramatic change occurs as life assumes a fresh sense of urgency. Many people start to realize how important support networks are at this point. Friends, family, and medical professionals turn into vital allies. Discussions turn to alternatives for therapy, the complexities of medical terminology, and making plans for the future. The foundation for future achievements is laid by acknowledging the importance of these relationships.

Another important stage is the start of treatment. For some, this involves surgery; for others, it involves radiation or chemotherapy. Every treatment plan has its own set of difficulties and successes. For example, celebrating the end of the first round of chemotherapy becomes a potent act of resistance to the illness. It's a concrete recognition of persevering in the face of adversity. Developing routines around these occasions frequently gives patients strength. What may have seemed like a lonely struggle can become a communal celebration of life with a modest get-together to mark the conclusion of a treatment cycle.

Treatment-induced physical changes can influence survivors' perceptions of their bodies. Scars, weight changes, and hair loss frequently inspire new ways of expressing oneself. This change is welcomed by many survivors as evidence of their journey. Regaining control over one's body might be symbolized by shaving one's head or going for a daring new hairstyle. In addition to enduring treatment, survivors must redefine courage and beauty in the midst of hardship. Every option, from the color of a new wig to the decision to forgo one, can mark a turning point in one's self-acceptance.

As time goes on, the emphasis can move from short-term care to long-term wellbeing and health. Regular examinations and scans turn into signs of hope. Every unambiguous test result is reason for jubilation and a brief reprieve. Survivors frequently thank themselves for these minor triumphs, understanding that each year and each clear scan adds to their continuous story of resiliency. These milestones are often shared on social media platforms, which enable people to engage with a larger community. A spirit of camaraderie is fostered when posts commemorating anniversaries of diagnosis or recovery serve as rays of hope for those going through similar experiences.

It is impossible to undervalue the importance of advocacy in the survivorship process. Sharing their stories, whether through writing, public speaking, or taking part in awareness campaigns, gives many people a sense of purpose. Through storytelling, survivors can transform their experiences into effective change agents, frequently signaling a turning point from survival to advocacy. They motivate those still fighting, educate others about the value of early detection, and increase awareness of breast cancer by sharing their own stories. Advocacy milestones have the potential to have just as much of an impact as personal ones. Giving a speech at a gathering or helping to raise money for research might give survivors the confidence to take control of their stories.

In order to successfully navigate the survivorship journey, support groups are essential. Many people view these organizations as secure places where they may talk about their successes, anxieties, and experiences. Making connections with people who are aware of the subtleties of this path can be a huge accomplishment in and of itself. In these groups, commemorating anniversaries strengthens the idea that no one is fighting their war alone and promotes a sense of togetherness. Sharing inspirational tales of recovery and hope can inspire others to stand together and seek support.

Physical activity also turns into a potent emblem of resiliency. Important milestones can be reached by taking part in activities like walks, runs, or bicycle challenges. A sense of survival is strengthened by the friendships formed during these occasions. For many, finishing a breast cancer awareness charity race is a celebration of their journey, resiliency, and community more than just a physical accomplishment. The personal journey is further entwined with larger social endeavors through these actions, which frequently result in increased awareness and financing for research.

Celebrating surviving milestones also requires spirituality and personal development. Some people undergo significant personal changes as a result of reevaluating their priorities after battling cancer. A stronger bond with oneself, a change in viewpoints, or even a renewed enthusiasm for life could be sparked by this adventure. The survivor's experience is enhanced by commemorating significant achievements in personal development, such as taking up new interests, practicing mindfulness, or cultivating connections. These instances show how self-discovery and healing are intertwined, enabling people to face life with newfound energy.

After therapy is finished, the road continues. Being a survivor requires constant introspection and celebration. Every day, week, or year that goes by offers a chance to recognize the fortitude required to overcome the obstacles. Whether through introspection, art, or community service, survivors frequently find themselves commemorating anniversaries with thankfulness. By cultivating a sense of calm and gratitude for life, these activities enable survivors to completely enjoy every moment.

Hope, strength, and awareness are woven into a complicated tapestry that represents the road of eradicating breast cancer. Every significant event, from the initial stages of diagnosis to the in-depth exploration of personal advocacy, adds to the compelling story of perseverance. In addition to honoring the individual's experience, commemorating these occasions benefits the larger community and leaves a legacy of resilience and consciousness for coming generations. With every step, the journey transforms from one of survival to one of purposeful, meaningful living and a deep sense of community.

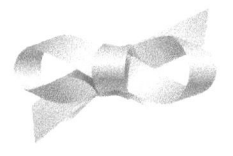

Resolving Persistent Adverse Effects

THERAPY FOR BREAST cancer frequently results in a complicated web of experiences that go well beyond the initial diagnosis and therapy. Long-lasting adverse effects are common for survivors and might continue long after active therapy ends. These impacts, which impact both mental and physical health, might differ greatly. Fostering resilience and improving the quality of life for individuals who have walked this difficult route need acknowledging and treating these enduring effects.

One of the most regularly reported adverse effects is fatigue, which frequently persists even after chemotherapy or radiation treatment is finished. This weariness is more than just a feeling of exhaustion; it may permeate every area of life and make even easy chores seem difficult. According to some survivors, it is a constant feeling of fatigue that interferes with their capacity to actively participate in everyday tasks or spend quality time with loved ones. A diversified strategy is needed to address this tiredness. A more balanced energy level can be achieved by gradually increasing physical activity while maintaining proper rest and nourishment. Yoga and meditation are examples of mindfulness exercises that may be beneficial in reducing stress and fostering serenity.

A variety of emotional reactions can be influenced by physical changes, frequently brought on by surgery or hormone treatments. Changes in body image might cause self-consciousness, uncertainty, or emotions of loss. A lot of survivors struggle with how these changes impact their relationships and sense of self. Participating in counseling or support groups can offer a secure setting for people to communicate their emotions and establish connections with like-minded others. In addition to helping to normalize the emotional upheaval that often accompany physical changes, these contacts frequently promote a sense of community.

Long after treatment, cognitive side effects, popularly known as "chemo brain," may still be present. Survivors may have trouble focusing, remembering things, or processing information. This mental haze can make everyday living even more frustrating and anxious, especially in academic or professional contexts. Cognitive rehabilitation exercises and memory aides like calendars, lists, or applications that improve focus and organization are ways to lessen these impacts. Over time, cognitive talents can also be sharpened by partaking in stimulating activities like reading, solving puzzles, or acquiring new skills.

Following breast cancer therapy, emotional health frequently suffers. Fears of recurrence and uncertainty about one's health can cause anxiety and sadness. Survivors may struggle with a shifted perspective, which can rise to existential concerns about life, meaning, and aspirations for the future. Professional therapy or counseling can offer vital support by providing a framework for processing these feelings as well as coping mechanisms. Furthermore, journaling is a useful tool for self-expression since it can assist people in expressing their ideas and emotions.

For those who have survived breast cancer, the social environment might change significantly. Because some others may find it difficult to comprehend the survivor's journey or the aftereffects of treatment, relationships with family and friends may change. Some relationships may grow stronger for survivors, while others may deteriorate or end completely. Discussing wants and feelings can help close understanding gaps and preserve relationships, so open communication is crucial. Loved ones' support can be crucial to recovery, offering survivors both practical help and emotional support as they adjust to their new normal.

Another important factor in controlling persistent side effects is nutrition. Following treatment, many survivors discover that their nutritional requirements vary as a result of modifications in taste, digestion, or energy levels. Lean meats, whole grains, fruits, and vegetables make constitute a balanced diet that helps promote healing and improve general health. Some people might find it helpful to speak with an oncology-focused nutritionist to customize their diet to suit their unique requirements and preferences. Trying out new dishes and recipes can help rekindle passion for cooking and eating, making meals enjoyable rather than a job.

Healing is frequently a nonlinear process, with survivors going through phases of advancement and regression. In this process, patience turns into a useful friend. The urge to "get back to normal" as soon as possible might be lessened by acknowledging that having ups and downs is normal. A greater comprehension of one's own resilience and adaptability may result from accepting the idea of a new normal. A more optimistic attitude can be produced by acknowledging and appreciating minor accomplishments along the way, such as finishing a project, getting back in touch with a friend, or just taking in a beautiful day.

Advocacy and awareness can strengthen survivors as they continue their journey. Many decide to tell their tales, adding to the broader discussion about breast cancer and its consequences. This advocacy can take many different forms, such as volunteering for groups that support breast cancer, supporting research initiatives, or taking part in awareness campaigns. In addition to giving people a feeling of purpose, interacting with others in the community demystifies the experience for others who have not yet encountered such difficulties.

It can also be advantageous to incorporate alternative therapies into a post-treatment routine. Certain physical symptoms may be reduced by techniques like acupuncture, massage, or aromatherapy, which also encourage emotional and physical well-being. Many survivors discover that these holistic methods can improve their general sense of balance and health by supplementing traditional therapies.

·· ❦ ··

Prioritizing self-care is crucial for survivors as they navigate the challenges of life after breast cancer. Making time for enjoyable and relaxing activities can be a very effective way to combat stress. A sense of agency and enjoyment can be restored by pursuing one's interests, whether it be through hobbies, time spent in nature, or just watching a beloved movie or book.

The experience of each survivor is distinct and influenced by a variety of elements, including as personal history, support networks, and coping strategies. Although there is no one-size-fits-all method for dealing with persistent side effects, a more fulfilling and empowered life after breast cancer can be achieved by cultivating a support network, investigating different coping mechanisms, and accepting the experience.

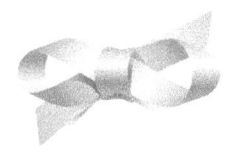

Getting Back into Everyday Life

ALTHOUGH THERE MAY be difficulties at every stage of this reintegration process, there are also chances for development and rejuvenation. Resilience, flexibility, and frequently a reinterpretation of what "normal" implies are necessary for the return to normalcy.

Resuming everyday habits can be intimidating in the beginning. Many survivors experience long-lasting physical side effects from radiation, chemotherapy, or surgery. For instance, fatigue may last even after the course of treatment is over. This weariness isn't just physical; it also includes emotional weariness from coping with the disease's psychological effects. Making self-care a priority becomes crucial throughout this period. Individuals can balance their energy levels with daily obligations by acknowledging their personal limits. A plan that incorporates relaxation, modest exercise, and time for introspection can help people feel in control even in the middle of chaos.

During and after therapy, social interactions frequently experience substantial changes. During the diagnostic and treatment stages, friends and family may come together to support a loved one, but when the immediate crisis has gone, the relationships may shift. It is possible for survivors to struggle with emotions of miscommunication or loneliness. Friends may avoid or act uneasy when discussing the experience since they are unsure of how to handle it. It's critical that people express their needs and feelings honestly. The gap between survivors and their loved ones can be closed by sharing experiences, whether in casual discussions or support groups. Stronger bonds and a greater understanding can result from this conversation.

Workplaces can add another level of difficulty. After a long break, some people might be going back to occupations that have seemed strange, while others might think about changing careers entirely. After cancer, the dynamics of the workplace can also change. It's possible for survivors to advocate for accommodations that meet their evolving requirements. It's critical to approach these discussions with confidence and clarity, highlighting the ways in which these changes can help the individual as well as the company overall.

In this reintegration process, balancing emotional well-being is essential. Survivors frequently feel a variety of feelings, ranging from relief and thankfulness to sadness and dread. Physical well-being, social support, and personal coping mechanisms are just a few of the variables that might impact this emotional terrain. Therapy or mindfulness exercises can assist people in navigating these emotional surges. Methods like writing, meditation, or even art therapy can offer a way to process and express oneself. These techniques foster a sense of action and empowerment in addition to helping with emotional regulation.

Another important component of reintegration is creating new routines that are consistent with personal beliefs. People frequently come away from their experiences with a fresh outlook on life, which leads them to reevaluate their priorities. This could show up as a dedication to leading a better lifestyle that includes regular exercise, a well-balanced diet, or mindfulness exercises. These lifestyle adjustments can promote long-term wellbeing and foster a sense of purpose. To further enhance their everyday lives, survivors may take up new interests or volunteer opportunities that align with their passions.

Reintegrating into regular life might also be aided by education and awareness of breast cancer. Sharing their experiences, spreading awareness, or promoting cancer support and research are all ways that many survivors find meaning in their work. Getting involved in the community can help you connect with people who have been through similar things. Engaging in activities such as walks or runs, giving speeches at neighborhood organizations, or using social media can turn individual experiences into more widespread knowledge. As survivors discover support and friendship in the community, this involvement can be a source of courage and healing.

A wide range of emotions can be evoked by revisiting physical settings. Going back to locations that were meaningful before the diagnosis, like parks, favorite cafes, or even well-known districts, can evoke thoughts and memories. Every visit can highlight the road that has been taken and act as a reminder of resiliency and personal development. But these locations can also make you feel depressed or anxious. It's important to handle these situations gently, letting oneself feel whatever comes up without passing judgment. These events can be made more manageable by creating a plan for handling them, such as attending with friends who are encouraging or practicing self-soothing methods.

After treatment, follow-up consultations and health examinations become essential parts of everyday life. These visits offer structure and reassurance, but they can also cause worry. Developing a rapport with medical professionals might increase survivors' sense of security by enabling them to freely express their worries and ask for advice. The focus can be changed from dread to proactive involvement in one's health journey by using these appointments as chances for empowerment and education.

Support networks are essential during this shift. A combination of official and informal support is frequently beneficial to survivors. Peer support groups, community services, and professional counseling can all provide priceless support. In the meanwhile, friends and family can offer equally important practical and emotional support. Creating a strong network of professional and personal connections promotes resilience and acts as a safety net in difficult times.

Chapter 6

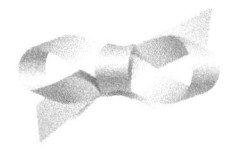

Awareness and Advocacy

In the battle against breast cancer, advocacy and awareness are essential pillars that provide a means for people and communities to come together in support of a shared goal. They act as rays of strength and hope, shedding light on the frequently difficult and depressing path taken by persons afflicted by this illness. Beyond just statistics, the stories surrounding breast cancer capture individual experiences, group resiliency, and shared narratives.

Advocacy is greatly aided by grassroots efforts, which enable people to share their experiences. Testimonies from real people can give the data a human face and inspire action by establishing an emotional bond. By inspiring others to speak up, these stories increase public awareness of early detection and the value of routine tests. These narratives are used by organizations devoted to breast cancer activism to inform and uplift communities. In order to demystify the illness and encourage preventative health measures, they plan conferences, workshops, and seminars.

To reach larger audiences, awareness campaigns frequently make use of a variety of media platforms. Social media sites have become essential resources for information sharing and community building. Innovative initiatives that use hashtags and viral challenges have the potential to become viral very rapidly, turning personal stories into compelling calls to action. In addition to educating people, these movements promote dialogue around breast health, creating an environment where people feel comfortable sharing their stories and worries.

One cannot stress the importance of education in raising awareness. Many people are ignorant of the fundamentals of breast cancer, such as its symptoms, risk factors, and available treatments. These gaps can be filled by educational initiatives in community centers, companies, and schools that offer useful knowledge that enables people to take charge of their health. Workshops conducted by medical experts can provide people the skills they need to identify possible signs and successfully navigate the healthcare system.

Additionally, advocacy influences healthcare access and research funding through its intersections with legislation and policy. More significant support for research projects and better access to screening and treatment can result from including politicians in conversations about breast cancer. In order to make their views heard, grassroots organizations might organize petitions and rallies to inspire community people to support change. At the municipal, state, and federal levels, this coordinated effort has the potential to significantly alter the way that breast cancer is addressed.

Another crucial component of managing the breast cancer experience is having strong community support networks. Support groups give people a place to interact, exchange stories, and offer support to one another. By letting people know they are not alone in their challenges, these groups can help them feel like they belong. Many groups offer tools and information about coping mechanisms, financial aid, and treatment choices in addition to emotional support.

Healthcare practitioners are essential to lobbying and awareness-raising as well. Results can be greatly impacted by their dedication to educating patients and their families. Social workers, nurses, and oncologists can offer crucial information regarding side effects, treatment alternatives, and lifestyle modifications. Additionally, by providing tools like counseling and support services, they can help patients navigate the emotional terrain of receiving a cancer diagnosis. Better health outcomes can result from healthcare practitioners empowering individuals to actively participate in their care through open communication.

The convergence of advocacy and technology in recent years has created new channels for raising awareness. People can now obtain information and support more easily thanks to telehealth services and mobile applications. By enabling connections across geographical borders, virtual communities help people who are facing comparable difficulties to feel more united. Social media groups and online forums can act as lifelines by providing immediate support and guidance from people who have been through similar experiences.

Creativity and the arts have also grown to be effective advocacy strategies for breast cancer. Through their platforms, artists and makers have raised awareness, frequently fusing personal stories with more general themes about the value of early detection and support. Digital information, performances, and art displays can all spark viewers' interest and comprehension by provoking thought-provoking dialogue. People may glimpse the faces behind the numbers by using this innovative method to humanize the statistics.

Furthermore, intersectionality in breast cancer advocacy highlights how critical it is to acknowledge the variety of experiences that those impacted by the disease have. People's perceptions and experiences with breast cancer are influenced by their cultural, financial, and geographic backgrounds. Outreach that is more inclusive and successful can result from adjusting advocacy initiatives to accommodate these differences. Advocates are better equipped to create messages that speak to the people who are most impacted when they have a thorough understanding of the particular difficulties that different groups experience.

Another important factor in the advocacy environment is survivorship. Honoring survivors' stories not only pays tribute to their experiences but also gives hope to those who are still fighting the illness. Initiatives conducted by survivors can encourage others to look for support and assistance, highlighting the value of community and resilience. Events like awareness walks and survivor parades bring people together in a common goal of eradicating breast cancer and serve as potent reminders of resilience in the face of hardship.

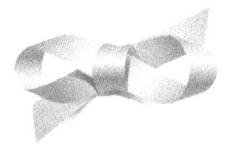

Telling Your Story: Giving Others Strength

A tapestry of experiences that can change a person's viewpoint and redefine relationships is frequently present during the breast cancer journey. Not only can telling your story about this journey help you heal yourself, but it can also encourage others who might be walking a similar path. Stories of breast cancer survivors' struggles and victories can strike a deep chord, fostering a sense of camaraderie and connection among people facing similar obstacles.

Sharing your story provides a special opportunity to draw attention to the range of feelings that come with receiving a breast cancer diagnosis. Every person has a unique experience that is influenced by their resilience, support networks, and circumstances. You can bring attention to the frequently unsaid anxieties, hardships, and victories that many people face by revealing the complexities of your experience. Others may find solace in this unvarnished sincerity, which serves as a reminder that they are not the only ones experiencing feelings of vulnerability and uncertainty.

Additionally, narrative can be a very effective way to raise awareness. The understanding of breast cancer becomes increasingly complex as more stories are shared. Awareness flourishes in personal accounts that emphasize the effects of this illness on people and their loved ones; it transcends data and medical classifications. Hearing a tale that resonates with one's own experience might lead to discussions regarding diagnosis, therapy, and emotional support that might not have otherwise taken place.

Sharing personal experiences not only increases awareness but also gives others the confidence to ask for assistance, speak up for their health, and make wise decisions. When given a diagnosis, many people may find it difficult to express their worries or inquiries. It might serve as a model for others to share their own feelings when they hear someone else voice their worries and fears. People with breast cancer are encouraged to embrace their voice and speak up for their needs because it fosters an atmosphere where vulnerability is greeted with understanding.

Additionally, sharing might act as a spark for the development of a community. Making connections with people who have gone through similar things gives many people comfort and helps them build support systems that offer practical, emotional, and even spiritual support. Support groups, neighborhood gatherings, and social media platforms can all help to build these relationships. By sharing their personal tales, people can encourage others to do the same, fostering a supportive and united community.

Breast cancer affects friends, family, and communities in addition to the individual. When people tell their stories, they shed light on the experiences of others around them. During this journey, friends, parents, and partners frequently bear their own problems, and sharing can provide them a chance to communicate their feelings and worries. By encouraging empathy and compassion, this group storytelling strengthens the ties that bind loved ones together through trying times.

Hope can also be sparked by tales of resiliency and survival. Hearing about someone's experience overcoming medication side effects and emotional obstacles can provide hope in a world that is frequently ruled by fear and uncertainty. It can inspire people who have just received a diagnosis to picture a strong, determined future. These kinds of stories serve as a reminder that even amid the most dire circumstances, people may find healing, development, and a new outlook on life.

Furthermore, exchanging experiences can demythologize the intricacies of medical care. The emotional toll of managing healthcare, the confusing array of alternatives, and the complexities of medical jargon can be too much to handle. By providing information about what to anticipate throughout therapy, the value of second opinions, and the necessity of mental health care, personal tales can help to dissolve these barriers. Others may be better equipped to handle their healthcare journeys with more assurance and comprehension because to these shared experiences.

Additionally, telling stories might help people feel more in control of their lives. While dealing with decisions that can feel overwhelming and burdensome, people with breast cancer may feel as though they have lost control. By telling their story, people can regain their sense of agency and turn a passive experience into an active one. It gives people the ability to take charge of their story and mold it to fit their preferences and ideals.

Another way to leave a legacy is via stories. For many people, living with breast cancer means more than just surviving; it means thriving and making a difference in the world. People can encourage future generations to address their health with awareness and bravery by sharing their personal journeys. It sows the seeds of understanding and information in a wider community, which may change the way future patients see their own experiences.

The effect of narrative can also be increased by using creative components. Writing, poetry, and art can offer more levels of expression, enabling people to communicate their experiences in distinctive ways. These artistic endeavors can serve as therapeutic tools, assisting people in processing their feelings and motivating others in the process.

The ability to connect is ultimately what gives stories their power. It can create a common area for empathy and understanding by bridging gaps between various backgrounds, cultures, and experiences. These tales can provide a sense of acceptance, support, and validation in the setting of breast cancer. People honor their own experiences and add to a communal narrative that highlights hope, courage, and perseverance when they decide to share their story.

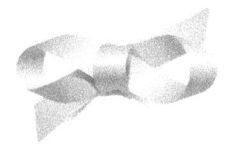

Getting Around Healthcare Systems and Getting Care

IT CAN BE VERY DIFFICULT to navigate the several healthcare systems after you have been diagnosed with breast cancer. In their quest for rehabilitation, patients frequently have to navigate a plethora of options, rules, and procedures, each of which could be a challenge. For individuals affected by breast cancer, knowing how to navigate these systems and finding a support network can have a big impact on their experience and results.

Getting a primary care physician or oncologist is frequently the initial step in this process. It is crucial to find a physician who shares the patient's values and needs in addition to having the necessary experience. Building strong relationships with the medical staff creates a space where patients feel free to express their worries, pose inquiries, and go over available treatments. Finding a doctor who is willing to take the time to discuss diagnoses, treatment options, and possible side effects should be a top priority for patients.

Having access to reliable information is crucial when dealing with breast cancer. It can be discouraging and perplexing for patients to be inundated with medical jargon and treatment processes. Advocacy groups offer helpful resources, including instructional materials that explain medical terminology and describe treatment options. Instead of being passive beneficiaries of care, these resources enable patients to take an active role in their treatment.

With its many different coverage plans, referral requirements, and insurance complexity, the healthcare system itself may be a labyrinth. A crucial part of getting care is understanding insurance coverage.

Patients need to become acquainted with their plan, knowing what operations, treatments, and prescription drugs are covered. With this information, unforeseen out-of-pocket costs during treatment can be avoided. Insurance navigators, who are frequently provided by hospitals or charitable groups, can help patients comprehend their benefits and figure out how to get the most out of their policy.

Community health initiatives help fill care gaps for those with low incomes. These initiatives frequently offer diagnostic imaging, screenings, and even treatment choices for no cost or at a reduced cost. In order to prevent access to care from becoming a barrier in the fight against breast cancer, organizations such as the American Cancer Society and neighborhood non-profits provide patient-specific support services. Financial advisors are also available at many hospitals to help people look into financial aid and assistance programs.

Another major barrier may be transportation, especially for people who live in rural areas. Patients without dependable transportation may not be able to make follow-up appointments or regular therapy sessions. Telehealth has become a useful tool that enables patients to communicate with medical professionals from a distance. Access to care can be improved by this innovation, especially for people who would find it difficult to travel for in-person sessions. Telehealth provides a practical option for consultations, follow-ups, and treatment plan talks, but it cannot replace every component of cancer care.

It is impossible to overestimate the emotional toll of receiving a breast cancer diagnosis. A patient's capacity to manage their medical journey may be impacted by the psychological effects. Online and in-person support groups provide essential emotional support by connecting patients with like-minded individuals. These relationships can promote a feeling of belonging and community, which lessens the loneliness of the journey. Additionally, oncology-focused mental health specialists can offer guidance and support, assisting patients in coping with anxiety, despair, and other emotional difficulties that may surface after treatment.

The way that people experience healthcare is greatly influenced by advocacy. In the healthcare system, patients ought to feel empowered to speak up for their needs and choices. This can involve seeking second opinions, looking for clinical trial prospects, and having discussions about cutting-edge therapy alternatives. Additionally, breast cancer advocacy groups put up a lot of effort to change healthcare policy in an effort to increase access to care and eradicate inequities. Patients and advocates may demand improved access and quality of care for everyone by banding together and enacting change.

Another essential component of navigating healthcare systems is cultural competence. Language hurdles and cultural variations in health attitudes and practices are two particular difficulties that patients from varied origins may face while trying to receive care. In order to guarantee that every patient receives fair and suitable treatment, healthcare professionals must make an effort to recognize and honor these distinctions. To ensure that no one is left behind in the healthcare journey, bilingual staff, culturally appropriate materials, and community outreach initiatives can all assist close these gaps.

For many people with breast cancer, clinical trials are a ray of hope because they provide access to innovative medicines that might not be generally accessible just yet. Navigating the clinical trial landscape, however, can be challenging. Patients should talk to their healthcare practitioners about the possibility of participating in a trial, taking into account things like eligibility requirements, possible advantages, and related risks. Additionally, clinical trial navigators can help patients identify studies that fit their unique diagnosis and treatment requirements and explain their options.

Continuity of care becomes more crucial as patients move through their treatment process. All facets of a patient's health are taken care of by coordinating communication between specialists, primary care physicians, and mental health specialists. Care coordination can also lessen the possibility of fragmented care, in which patients might get lost because of poor follow-up or misunderstandings. Patients ought to push for an all-encompassing care strategy that incorporates suggestions from all pertinent medical professionals.

The journey continues once therapy is over. Plans for survivorship care are crucial resources for negotiating the post-treatment environment. These plans specify the required follow-up care, recurrence monitoring, and methods for preserving general health and wellbeing. Patients can take control of their health as they adjust to life following treatment with the help of a well-designed survivorship care plan.

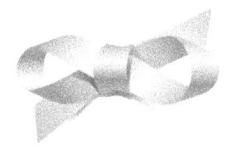

Keeping Up to Date: Advances, Prevention, and Research

Research on breast cancer covers a wide range of topics, such as genetics, early detection, and new therapeutic developments. With the discovery of genes like BRCA1 and BRCA2, the research of genetic predisposition has become much more popular in recent years. Genetic testing is necessary because women who have mutations in these genes are significantly more likely to develop breast cancer. Knowing one's genetic composition might enable people to make well-informed decisions regarding their health, including proactive steps like enhanced screening procedures or preventive mastectomy.

A key component of preventing breast cancer is routine mammograms, which enable early discovery when the condition is most curable. As mammography recommendations have changed, health organizations increasingly support customized screening programs based on risk factors. Women who have genetic alterations or a family history of breast cancer, for instance, would be urged to begin testing sooner. This individualized strategy emphasizes how crucial it is to understand and educate people about their unique risk factors.

The risk of breast cancer is greatly influenced by lifestyle decisions in addition to genetics. The connection between nutrition, exercise, and cancer prevention is still being investigated. Maintaining a healthy weight and lowering the risk of breast cancer can be achieved with a balanced diet full of fruits, vegetables, and whole grains as well as regular exercise. Healthy living initiatives, such nutrition classes and community fitness programs, provide people the power to take control of their health.

Hormone replacement treatment (HRT) has been the focus of much research in the field of preventive. Although HRT can help with menopausal symptoms, research suggests that long-term use may increase the risk of breast cancer. Because of this intricacy, patients and healthcare professionals must have educated conversations to balance the risks and benefits. Women can make decisions that are in line with their health priorities when they stay up to date on new information.

The patient experience has changed as a result of technological developments in breast cancer detection and therapy. For example, digital mammography provides better image quality and more accurate abnormality detection. Additionally, because it offers a more thorough image of breast tissue, breast MRI has become a useful tool for high-risk women. These advances highlight how important it is to stay up to date on the most recent advancements in screening technology.

Furthermore, patient outcomes have greatly improved as a result of developments in treatment approaches. When compared to conventional chemotherapy, targeted medicines like trastuzumab (Herceptin) have improved survival rates and reduced side effects, completely changing the way HER2-positive breast cancer is treated. Immunotherapy, which uses the body's immune system to fight cancer cells, is also becoming more and more popular as a viable strategy. Patients must be aware of these treatment alternatives in order to discuss individualized treatment plans and have meaningful interactions with their healthcare professionals.

Another way that patients can keep informed and help improve the research on breast cancer is by taking part in clinical studies. Clinical trials are crucial for evaluating novel treatments, comprehending the course of diseases, and finding creative preventative strategies. In addition to having access to state-of-the-art therapies, patients who take part in these trials also have a significant influence on how others will be treated in the future. Patients may feel more empowered to think about solutions that fit their situation if they are aware of ongoing scientific studies.

For people navigating the difficulties of breast cancer, advocacy groups and support networks are vital resources. These organizations offer instructional programs, support groups that promote community and connection, and information on nearby services. Feelings of uncertainty and loneliness can be reduced by interacting with people who have gone through similar things. Social media and online platforms have also become effective means of spreading personal narratives and increasing awareness, giving voice to those who are traveling similar paths.

Managing breast cancer requires a strong sense of mental and emotional health. Patients who participate in supportive therapies, such counseling or support groups, report higher quality of life and maybe better treatment outcomes, according to research. As patients and their families deal with the emotional difficulties brought on by a breast cancer diagnosis, it is crucial that they remain aware of available mental health options.

In order to inform the public about breast cancer, its risk factors, and the significance of early detection, awareness campaigns are essential. Information is spread through campaigns like Breast Cancer Awareness Month, which motivate people to prioritize routine tests and self-examinations. Walks and fundraisers are examples of community events that bring people together in the battle against breast cancer by fostering a sense of purpose and solidarity. These advertisements have the potential to be potent reminders of the tenacity and strength of the disease's victims as a whole.

The field of breast cancer prevention, detection, and therapy is growing more complex as science advances. Being informed enables people to make decisions that are consistent with their unique circumstances and values while navigating this journey with confidence and knowledge. Knowledge is still an essential tool in the pursuit of awareness and empowerment, whether it be by investigating new treatment options, adopting a healthy lifestyle, or comprehending inherited hazards.

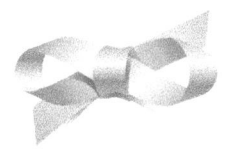

Conclusion

RECEIVING A BREAST cancer diagnosis can be devastating for the patient and their loved ones. Everybody's path is different, with feelings that fluctuate like the tide. Comprehending the terrain of this encounter can offer some solace.

The basis for action is awareness. When faced with the illness for the first time, many people may feel bewildered or alone. This feeling of isolation may result from a lack of knowledge about breast cancer in general as well as the resources that are available. Support groups, community gatherings, and educational initiatives are crucial in breaking the taboo. They build relationships and promote communication that can help dispel the stigma associated with the diagnosis.

Getting around the medical system can be difficult at times. The experience can seem overwhelming due to the abundance of specialists, treatment options, and medical jargon. Asking inquiries and gathering facts are essential, but it's important to speak up for oneself. Interacting with medical professionals helps people feel in control of what can otherwise seem like a chaotic circumstance. Every appointment is a chance to get questions answered and learn about the future.

One of the most important aspects of the journey is emotional support. Making connections with people who have gone through similar things can help people feel less alone. In-person or online, support groups provide a secure environment for sharing hopes, anxieties, and everything in between. People form relationships through sharing stories, which serves as a reminder that they are not fighting this battle alone. Vulnerability is a strength, and being vulnerable can result in unforeseen friendships and a feeling of belonging.

Friends and family can be a great asset. Loved ones, however, could find it difficult to understand the psychological and physical toll that illness takes. It is crucial to communicate; expressing wants can open the door to more meaningful relationships. They can provide useful assistance, including preparing meals or going to appointments with people. Even though they are modest, these actions have a big impact on reducing stress and building resilience.

Keeping a sense of hope becomes crucial during the journey. This does not entail denying unpleasant feelings or acting as though nothing is wrong. Instead, it entails facing anxieties while maintaining an optimistic outlook. Concentrating on minor successes might change viewpoints. These moments, whether it's a successful test or a pain-free day, can act as moorings when things become rough.

Self-care and mindfulness techniques provide strategies for coping with the emotional ups and downs of cancer treatment. Inner serenity can be developed through practices like journaling, yoga, and meditation. In the midst of the chaos, finding delight in hobbies, the outdoors, or the arts can help restore a feeling of normalcy. Establishing a habit that incorporates these techniques is essential for building grounding and resilience.

Navigating the intricacies of treatment requires good physical health. A healthy diet, consistent exercise, and enough sleep all support general wellbeing. Every decision one makes can seem like a step toward empowerment and a return to bodily control. It's not always simple, particularly when side effects from therapy appear, but getting advice from dietitians or fitness professionals can offer specialized assistance.

The field of breast cancer treatment is always changing. Medical advancements like immunotherapy and targeted medicines open up new therapeutic options. Keeping up with the most recent findings can help people feel more in control of their lives. Access to innovative therapies may also be provided by taking part in clinical trials. This gives some people hope for a better future.

It is impossible to overstate the importance of creativity in coping. Painting, writing, or music are all forms of artistic expression that provide comfort to many. This kind of self-expression gives people a strong emotional release and helps them understand their journey. When needed most, creativity can provide solace by igniting happiness and a sense of community.

It becomes clear how important balance is when one travels this route. Having both good and terrible days is normal. It is crucial to give oneself permission to feel the entire spectrum of emotions. Adopting this equilibrium can help people become more resilient and see the path ahead more clearly.

Participating in breast cancer awareness initiatives adds to a broader story. These programs enable people to take control of their health in addition to helping to finance research. Sharing personal accounts on social media or at neighborhood gatherings promotes candid conversations about breast health and lessens stigma. People can become champions by speaking up, encouraging others to give screenings and preventative measures top priority.

Being adaptable is essential when navigating the difficulties of breast cancer. Emotions might be erratic, plans can vary, and treatment procedures can alter. Over time, the ability to adjust to these changes is developed. People who are flexible in their thinking and behavior are able to gracefully negotiate uncertainty and transform obstacles into chances for personal development.

During difficult circumstances, including faith can be consoling. Many people find that their faith gives them courage and helps them get through difficult times. These activities, whether they involve prayer, meditation, or spending time in nature, can bring about a sense of calm. Examining one's spiritual beliefs might help one understand themselves better and find comfort in the face of adversity.

In the end, overcoming breast cancer serves as a tribute to the human spirit. Every person's journey is characterized by unique obstacles, victories, and revelations. Being strong means more than just fighting the illness; it also means having the fortitude to face anxieties, rely on support networks, and appreciate the beauty of life despite hardship.

Awareness of breast cancer continues to grow, learn, and connect throughout one's life after receiving a diagnosis. By sharing their experiences and cultivating a community based on compassion and understanding, those who travel this route become emissaries of hope. Deep changes can result from welcoming this trip with open arms, serving as a reminder to everyone that awareness, hope, and strength are all entwined in one continuous story.